Neurology

STUDENT NOTES

Neurology

Christopher N. Martyn MA DPhil MRCP
Clinical Scientist, MRC Environmental Epidemiology Unit,
Southampton General Hospital;
Honorary Senior Registrar in Neurology,
Wessex Neurological Centre, Southampton General Hospital, Southampton, UK

CHURCHILL LIVINGSTONE
EDINBURGH LONDON MELBOURNE AND NEW YORK 1989

CHURCHILL LIVINGSTONE
Medical Division of Longman Group UK Limited

Distributed in the United States of America by Churchill
Livingstone Inc., 1560 Broadway, New York, N.Y. 10036,
and by associated companies, branches and representatives
throughout the world.

First published 1989

ISBN 0-443-03307-2

British Library Cataloguing in Publication Data
Martyn, Christopher N.
  Neurology.
  1. Medicine. Neurology
  I. Title
  616.8

Library of Congress Cataloging in Publication Data
Martyn, Christopher N.
  Neurology/Christopher N. Martyn.
    p.   cm.—(Student notes)
  Bibliography: p.
  Includes index.
  1. Neurology. 2. Nervous system—Diseases. I. Title.
  II. Series.
  [DNLM: 1. Nervous System Diseases. WL 100 M3875n]
  RC346.M296   1989
  616.8—dc20
  DNLM/DLC
  for Library of Congress   89–7088
                                                    CIP

Produced by Longman Singapore Publishers (Pte) Ltd.
Printed in Singapore.

Preface

This book is intended to provide medical students with a short and practical introduction to clinical neurology. There are three sections: the first deals with taking a history and carrying out an examination of the nervous system, the second with radiological, electrophysiological and laboratory investigations and the third with the commoner diseases that affect the nervous system.

In a perceptive article published in the *British Medical Journal* several years ago on what was wrong with medical textbooks John Launer, then a medical student, argued that many authors failed to show enough sympathy with the inevitable ignorance of the beginner. As a student myself at the time the piece was written I agreed with him completely, and when writing this book I have tried to keep this point in mind. The emphasis throughout is on how to acquire the clinical skills needed for diagnosis and management. When writing about diseases of the nervous system I have concentrated on conditions which are important either because they are common or because they are treatable. Many of the rare syndromes which make neurology such a difficult subject for someone grappling with it for the first time are deliberately neglected. I have also assumed that most students will have forgotten a lot of what they were taught in their preclinical courses and, where it is needed to understand a part of the clinical examination or a feature of a disease, the relevant neuroanatomy and neurophysiology is explained.

Many people have encouraged and helped me to write this book. Dr Robin Sellar, consultant neuroradiologist at the Western General Hospital, Edinburgh, collaborated in the writing of the chapter on radiological investigation. Dr Brian Pentland and Dr Roger Cull made valuable comments on early drafts. Two Southampton medical students, Mary Lambert and Cathy Laird, read the book when it was nearing completion and tactfully drew my attention to points in the text where explanations were obscure or descriptions ambiguous. I am indebted to them all.

Southampton, 1989   C.N.M.

Contents

Taking a history and examining the nervous system

1. Taking a neurological history

Learning how to take an accurate medical history requires a lot of practice and reading about how to do it is no substitute for talking to patients. Just as you can't discover much about parachuting if you never leave the ground you can't learn much about history-taking unless you spend time at the bedside. Nonetheless, those just beginning clinical medicine may find some advice helpful.

When students first start seeing patients one of their main concerns is trying to remember all the questions that they are supposed to ask. This preoccupation encourages the belief that taking a history is no more than a matter of filling in a sort of notional questionnaire. It is certainly true that the patient's history must be taken in a systematic and comprehensive way. But this should not detract from the fact that history-taking needs to be an active intellectual process far removed from the method used by market researchers when they place ticks in boxes to record their victim's responses to rigidly worded questions.

Experienced physicians start to formulate tentative hypotheses about the diagnosis quite early on during an encounter with a patient. They are able to do this for two reasons. First, they can draw on their knowledge of which diseases commonly occur in people of the same age and sex as their patient. Second, they can discern a pattern in the symptoms that the patient describes which matches, more or less, what they know about a particular disease. Questions can then be directed in a way which will confirm or refute the initial idea. Often, of course, first thoughts about the diagnosis prove to be mistaken and it becomes necessary to take a new approach, but the point being emphasized is that successful history-taking demands alertness and vigorous thought from the history taker. He needs first to notice any diagnostic clues offered by the patient and then to phrase specific enquiries to follow them up.

3

Novices in the art of taking medical histories cannot expect always to be successful in reaching the right diagnosis. Deciding what is important and what should be ignored out of the rag-bag of facts that emerge when you start talking to a patient is not easy. Knowledge of the clinical features of diseases of the nervous system and experience of different ways in which these diseases present is necessary. Until you have gained this knowledge and experience the following scheme will help you structure your history taking. Try to use the headings as prompts for different lines of enquiry rather than as a catechism of questions to ask the patient.

SCHEME FOR TAKING A NEUROLOGICAL HISTORY

The presenting complaint

What is the reason that the patient has sought medical advice? If the symptoms have been present for some time why has he come now? Analyse the symptoms under the following headings.

Description of the nature and quality of the symptoms

What is the main problem? For example: pain, loss of function, weakness, sensory loss, disturbance of sphincter control. Are the symptoms getting better or worse?

Location

Which part of the body is affected?

Timing

When did the symptoms first start?
Was the onset sudden or gradual?
Are the symptoms constant or intermittent?
If the symptoms are intermittent, how long do they last?

Precipitating factors

What brings the symptoms on?

Exacerbating and relieving factors

What makes the symptoms better?
What makes them worse?

Associated features

Is there anything associated with the major symptoms?
 Ask specifically about:
episodes of loss of consciousness
blackouts and dizzy turns
problems with memory or concentration
speech problems
difficulty with chewing or swallowing
eyesight: visual acuity, diplopia and obscuration of vision
disturbance of sphincter control
loss of muscular power in limbs
difficulty in walking
sensory disturbance: numbness and paraesthesiae
headache

Medical history

Has the patient had any serious illness in the past? Has he ever been admitted to hospital? If so, what was the reason for admission? Ask patients with neurological symptoms if they have ever had a head injury severe enough to cause loss of consciousness.

Review of systems

A brief enquiry about major symptoms in the other organ systems should be made.

Family history

Special attention should be given to the family history because of the large number of neurological diseases that are familial or genetic. Enquire about the patient's siblings, including those who have died, parents and grandparents. Ask a general question to find out whether there are any diseases of the nervous system that run in the family.

Information from witnesses

Many neurological conditions involve loss of or alteration in consciousness or deterioration in memory or intellect. In these circumstances, it is very important to speak to relatives or other witnesses to get a reliable account of the patient's illness.

In conclusion

At the end of taking a history it may be helpful to ask the patient if anything important has been omitted or if there is anything he wants to add to the account he has given. This is a convenient time to ask about his own theories concerning his symptoms; he may reveal anxieties that need to be discussed later. It is a good practice to recapitulate the history back to the patient. This gives him a chance to correct or amplify certain points and allows him to be confident that you have understood his story properly.

EVALUATION OF THE HISTORY

It is worth considering some of the constraints that may prevent your patient from giving an entirely straightforward account of his illness. Many of these are obvious enough. For example, unless you have the misfortune to have a sick doctor as a patient, it is unlikely that he has the vocabulary to describe his symptoms and disability with precision. Any medical terms that he does employ are probably misused. You must be sure that you understand exactly what the patient means when he uses ambiguous terms like 'feeling dizzy' or 'blackout'. Even a word like 'numb', which you might think carried only one meaning, may be used idiosyncratically to describe loss of muscular strength rather than loss of sensation.

Although you should endeavour to allow the patient to explain his symptoms in his own words you will often need to follow up with supplementary questions in order to clarify exactly what is meant. Sometimes the sensation that the patient is trying to describe is so far outside the range of his experience that it becomes necessary to supply him with the right words to explain it. The aura of a temporal lobe attack for instance, is so strange that you may have to ask specific questions about olfactory hallucinations or sensations of déjà vu to help him communicate his feelings of altered perception. Beware though, of the dangers of biasing the evidence if you suggest words to the patient.

Another source of difficulty in interpreting a history occurs if the patient is embarrassed by his symptoms. Most adults are understandably reluctant to admit to loss of sphincter control or to confide the circumstances if the symptoms occurred during sexual intercourse. You should consider too, any consequences of the illness for the patient's livelihood; someone whose work involves driving or working with machinery may give a less than frank account of episodes of loss of consciousness.

Not much imagination is needed to realise that, however well they may conceal it, most patients are extremely anxious about their symptoms. You should try to explore the reasons for their anxiety. For example, a patient may consult you about headaches which he has had for a long time only because a friend or relative has recently died of a brain tumour. This sort of information is essential for successful management. Unless the explanation of the symptoms that you give to the patient takes account of his own worries and theories about his illness, he is unlikely to find it very convincing or reassuring.

2. The motor system

NEUROANATOMY AND NEUROPHYSIOLOGY

Any series of co-ordinated muscular movements, whether semi-automatic like walking, or more consciously controlled like playing a piano, depends on a complicated sequence of neural events in many parts of the brain and spinal cord. The allocation of one particular aspect of the control of muscle activity to one area of the nervous system, such as voluntary skilled movement to the primary motor cortex or co-ordination to the cerebellum, is an oversimplification. In clinical practice though, straightforward notions about the function of areas of the brain often serve well enough. You will find it more helpful to have a few simple but easily remembered concepts of the neural apparatus of the motor system than to know about the most up-to-date but complicated theories concerning, for example, subcortical motor programmes.

The next few pages provide a brief revision of the structure and function of those parts of the nervous system concerned with the control of muscle activity.

Cortical areas of motor control

The principal cortical area concerned with the control of skilled movements is located in the precentral gyrus (Fig. 2.1). The topographical organization of the primary motor cortex can be remembered by recalling the homunculus which Penfield derived from stimulating this strip of cortex and observing the movements that resulted (Fig. 2.2). Most of the motor axons that descend in the corticospinal tracts originate from this area. Others arise from areas of cortex both anterior and posterior to the primary motor strip.

The primary motor cortex is actually quite low down in the hierarchy of structures involved in motor control. It is, after all,

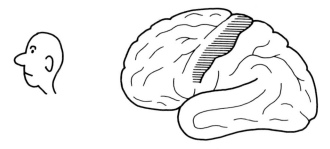

Fig. 2.1 The primary motor cortex is located in the precentral gyrus (shown hatched).

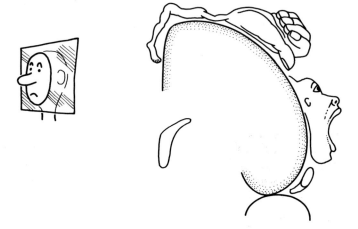

Fig. 2.2 The topographical organization of the motor cortex.

only a synapse or two away from the lower motor neurone, the final common pathway for activating muscle contraction. The primary motor cortex is certainly not the area of the brain in which the decision to make a voluntary movement is taken. You will meet patients whose difficulties with motor control arise, not because of paralysis or inco-ordination, but because they have lost the ability to formulate a strategy for carrying out a series of movements in the correct sequence. Such a patient, for example, may be unable to tie his shoe laces despite the absence of any weakness or loss of co-ordination. The lesion in this case is not in the primary motor cortex but in a part of the brain concerned with a higher level of motor control. This sort of problem with motor control is known as *apraxia* and is discussed further in Chapter 7.

The corticospinal tract

Nerve fibres from the primary motor cortex converge in a fan-like way through the corona radiata into the posterior limb of the internal capsule. The compact arrangement of the cortical motor outflow in the internal capsule is important because it means that even a small lesion there affects movements of the whole of the contralateral half of the body.

On each side of the brain the internal capsule is continuous with the cerebral peduncles—the main trunks of communication between cerebral hemispheres and brain stem. As they descend through the pons the fibre tracts of the corticospinal pathways become dispersed into small bundles but they converge again in the upper medulla to form the medullary pyramids. It is from these structures that the corticospinal tracts gain their alternative name of *pyramidal tracts*. At the lowest, most caudal part of the medulla, just above the foramen magnum, the fibres of the corticospinal tracts cross to the opposite side of the brain stem in the medullary decussation. Textbooks of neuroanatomy will inform you that about 10% of the fibres remain uncrossed, but neurologists rarely find this fact of clinical value.

After decussating, the corticospinal tracts lie in the lateral part of the spinal cord and remain in this position as they run caudally. At each segmental level axons turn medially to synapse with the cell body of the lower motor neurone in the anterior horn of the grey matter of the spinal cord. The lower motor neurone exits from the spinal cord by the ventral (anterior) root and joins with other motor neurones to form a peripheral motor nerve supplying skeletal muscle.

Some nerve fibres arising in the motor cortex cross in the brain stem above the main medullary decussation to synapse in the cranial nerve motor nuclei. The motor nuclei of the cranial nerves are collections of cell bodies of the lower motor neurones that form the peripheral part of the cranial nerves. Functionally, they are the equivalent of the cells in the anterior horns of the grey matter of the cord.

The anatomy of the corticospinal pathway is summarized in Figure 2.3.

Clinical features of lesions in the corticospinal pathway

The earliest sign of dysfunction in the motor cortex or corticospinal pathways is poor performance of skilled and fine repetitive

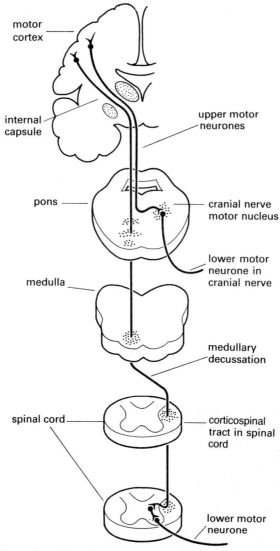

motor cortex

internal capsule

upper motor neurones

pons

cranial nerve motor nucleus

lower motor neurone in cranial nerve

medulla

medullary decussation

spinal cord

corticospinal tract in spinal cord

lower motor neurone

Fig. 2.3 The corticospinal pathway.

movements. This is usually most noticeable in the hands and fingers. More extensive lesions of the corticospinal tracts cause weakness; the extensor muscles of the upper limb and the flexor muscles of the lower limb are the most severely affected. Muscle tone is increased and tendon reflexes are pathologically brisk. The plantar response is extensor. The physiological explanation for the changes in muscle tone and tendon reflexes is discussed on page 19.

Whether the side of the body ipsilateral or contralateral to the lesion is affected depends on the site of the lesion. Damage in the cortex, internal capsule, midbrain or pons—anywhere, in fact, rostral to the medullary decussation—will result in a contralateral hemiparesis. If the lesion is below the medullary decussation in the spinal cord the ipsilateral side of the body is affected.

The extrapyramidal system

Neuroanatomists and physiologists complain that the term extrapyramidal system is unsatisfactory from both anatomical and functional viewpoints. They point out that the pyramidal system and the extrapyramidal system are closely interlinked by fibre connections and that the two systems should in no sense be considered as alternatives or rivals. Clinical neurologists, however, often use the term extrapyramidal system as convenient shorthand for the basal ganglia and related structures and this convention will be maintained here.

The major structures which constitute the extrapyramidal system are listed below:

1. basal ganglia:
   a. caudate nucleus
   b. putamen
   c. globus pallidus
   d. substantia nigra
   e. subthalamic nucleus
2. thalamus
3. red nucleus
4. vestibular nuclei.

The caudate nucleus and putamen are anatomically and functionally closely related and are sometimes referred to collectively as the striatum.

Recent work has identified some of the extremely complex pathways and transmitter systems linking these structures. The basal ganglia receive inputs from nearly the whole of the cerebral cortex and the thalamus and the substantia nigra. The major output of the basal ganglia is from the globus pallidus which projects, via the thalamus, to the motor cortex and back to the substantia

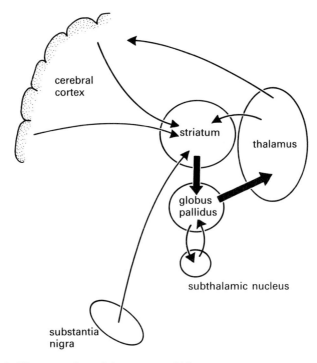

Fig. 2.4   The connections of the extrapyramidal system.

nigra. A simplified scheme of the interconnections of the extrapyramidal system is shown in Figure 2.4.

Despite increasing knowledge of the connections and neurotransmitters of the extrapyramidal system our understanding of how it actually works in the production and control of movement is still very limited and there is little to be gained by memorizing the details of these pathways. There is no doubt that the extrapyramidal structures play a vital role in the control of movement, but their precise function remains controversial. One idea is that, situated as they are between the thalamus—a structure that receives a huge afferent sensory input—and the cortex, they mediate in a dialogue between incoming sensory information and the motor cortex. They are involved perhaps, in deciding a strategy for movement and in initiating the complex motor patterns' with which we respond to sensory stimuli. Another view is that the extrapyramidal system is concerned with the storage and accessing of learned motor programmes.

Little is known about the functioning of the red nucleus and the vestibular nuclei in man. Evidence from animal experiments seems to indicate that the red nucleus and its descending spinal pathway are mainly concerned in the control of proximal limb musculature. The vestibular nuclei, as one would guess from their name, receive a major afferent input from the semicircular canals. They are probably involved in the control of axial and antigravity muscles, particularly those concerned with movement of the head.

Clinical features of disease of the extrapyramidal system

Disease of the extrapyramidal system is usually bilateral although there may be some asymmetry in the degree to which the two sides of the brain are affected. The descending extrapyramidal outflow is crossed so that in the rare cases of unilateral disease it is the contralateral side of the body which is affected.

Four main features characterize extrapyramidal disease:

1. difficulty in the initiation of movement (known as bradykinesia or hypokinesia)
2. disturbance of muscle tone
3. the appearance of involuntary movements
4. disturbance of posture.

Bradykinesia. The patient is slow to initiate and execute both voluntary and involuntary movements. His face is immobile and expressionless and he blinks only infrequently. He shuffles along with small steps instead of striding out and he loses associated movements such as swinging his arms when he walks and making hand gestures when he speaks.

Hypertonia. Muscle tone is usually increased in disorders of the extrapyramidal system. This increase is largely independent of the muscle stretch reflex so that when the limb is moved passively, an increased resistance is felt throughout the whole range of movement of the joint. To the examiner the sensation is like that of bending a lead pipe.

This pattern of increased muscle tone is known as *rigidity.* Contrast it with the *spasticity* found in lesions of the pyramidal tract where there is an initial high resistance to passive movement followed by a sudden 'give'; a phenomenon dependent on the presence of an overactive muscle stretch reflex.

Involuntary movements. A number of descriptive words are used to classify involuntary movements.

Athetosis refers to slow writhing movements of the distal parts of limbs, especially hands and fingers.

Chorea is a term that is derived from the Greek word meaning dance. It describes apparently random, unpredictable, sudden, jerky movements of the limbs or trunk.

Hemiballismus is the name given to sudden, violent, high amplitude movements of the limbs on one side of the body. The presence of hemiballismus usually indicates a lesion in the contralateral subthalamic nucleus.

Tremor is the commonest type of involuntary movement. Most people exhibit a high frequency low amplitude shakiness of the finger tips in times of stress. This is known as *physiological tremor* and should not be thought to indicate neurological disease. Tremor resulting from disease of the extrapyramidal system is more complex involving several different muscle groups. It is rather lower in frequency and higher in amplitude than physiological tremor. In Parkinson's disease, the commonest disorder of the extrapyramidal system, tremor often manifests itself as a rhythmic flexion and extension of the fingers coupled with a rotatory oscillation of the wrist. The phenomenon is still frequently described as a *pill rolling tremor* despite the fact that modern pharmaceutical technology has robbed the metaphor of its vividness.

Change in posture. A patient with Parkinson's disease stands in a characteristic flexed posture (see Fig. 2.7). Other diseases of the extrapyramidal system affect posture too. In the rare condition of progressive supranuclear palsy the neck muscles become rigid and the head is held in a retracted position. In cases of torsion dystonia the patient may hold himself in such a bizarre posture that a mistaken diagnosis of a psychiatric disorder rather than neurological disease is made.

The cerebellum

There are several theories about the way in which the cerebellum functions. Perhaps the most illuminating for the clinical neurologist is the hypothesis that it acts as a comparator. This model suggests that the cerebellum compares the command for muscle contraction issued by the motor cortex with the actual movement that results and detects any shortfall or overshoot in performance. The cerebellum receives two important inputs; one from the motor cortex, a copy, as it were, of the order for move-

ment sent down the corticospinal tract; the other is a proprioceptive input via the spinocerebellar pathways from muscle spindles,
tendon organs and joint position receptors. The incoming
proprioceptive information keeps the cerebellum immediately in-
formed about limb and trunk movement and any mismatch between intended and actual movement is computed. Information
about error in the execution of the movement is fed back to the
motor cortex allowing it to modify the signals being sent to the
active muscles.

The cerebellum consists of the two hemispheres and a midline
structure, the vermis. The hemispheres are concerned with limb
movements and the vermis with axial muscles and trunk movements. The pathways connecting cerebral cortex and propriocep-
tors with the cerebellum are shown in Figure 2.5. Each *cerebral*
hemisphere projects to the contralateral *cerebellar* hemisphere. By
contrast, proprioceptive information travels up the spinal cord in

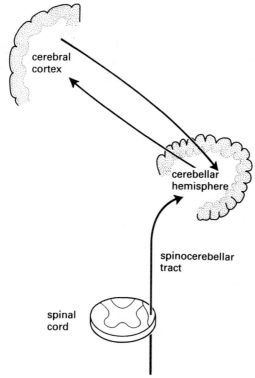

Fig. 2.5 Cerebellar connections.

the *uncrossed* spinocerebellar tracts to reach the ipsilateral cerebellar hemisphere. The main output of the cerebellum is back to the contralateral cerebral cortex. Lesions of a cerebellar hemisphere therefore result in difficulties in motor control that affect the ipsilateral side of the body.

Clinical features of disease of the cerebellum

Cerebellar dysfunction is manifested by inability to make smooth voluntary movements. The patient is clumsy and inco-ordinated, unable to produce the accurately timed sequence of individual muscle contractions necessary for precise movement. The general term for such unsteady and clumsy movements is *ataxia*. In addition, because rapid and co-ordinated movements of the lips, tongue and palate are affected, speech is slurred—a condition known as dysarthria. Disordered eye movements, most commonly nystagmus, may be present.

The tendon reflex

The anatomical basis of the monosynaptic spinal reflex arc mediating the tendon reflex is shown in Figure 2.6. A sudden increase in muscle length, produced at the bedside by a blow from the physician's hammer on the muscle's tendon, is detected by muscle spindles in the belly of the muscle. The resulting burst of afferent impulses rapidly ascends to the spinal cord along large myelinated sensory fibres. These fibres synapse with the lower motor neurones in the spinal cord and excite them to discharge a volley of efferent impulses which cause a brief muscle contraction.

The amplitude of this muscle contraction depends on the level of excitability of the motor neurone pool. Excitability is controlled by many descending influences from both pyramidal and extrapyramidal sources and from adjacent spinal segments. The overall influence from the higher centres is normally inhibitory. When a lesion in the corticospinal tract is present, lower motor neurones below the level of the lesion escape from the descending inhibitory traffic of nerve impulses and their excitability becomes set at a higher level. A burst of afferent impulses now discharges a greater number of lower motor neurones than before and this results in a stronger muscle contraction. Lesions of the corticospinal tracts therefore cause an exaggeration of the normal tendon reflex.

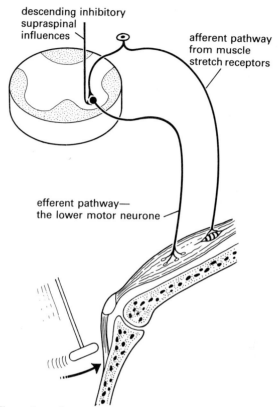

descending inhibitory
supraspinal
influences

afferent pathway
from muscle
stretch receptors

efferent pathway—
the lower motor neurone

Fig. 2.6   The tendon reflex.

However, eliciting a tendon reflex tests more than the level of excitability of the motor neurone pool and the integrity of synaptic transmission in the spinal cord because the reflex also depends on the functioning of proprioceptive afferent fibres and lower motor neurones. If disease of peripheral nerves or spinal roots is present, the reflex arc is interrupted and tendon reflexes are reduced or absent.

The increased muscle tone of the spastic pattern seen in disease of the corticospinal tracts (see page 12) is also the result of over-active muscle stretch reflexes. When the examiner flexes a joint to assess muscle tone, the initial stretch of the muscle reflexly produces active contraction. Because this reflex is exaggerated in lesions of the corticospinal tract resistance to passive flexion of a joint is increased. If the examiner persists, muscle tension continues to rise until a point is reached at which stretch receptors in the tendon, the Golgi tendon organs, are stimulated to fire. Afferents from tendon stretch receptors, in contrast to those from muscle stretch receptors, are strongly inhibitory to the motor neurone pool. The inhibitory influences from the tendon organs override the excitatory influences from the muscle spindles, active muscle contraction ceases and the examiner experiences a sudden 'give'—the *clasp-knife* phenomenon.

The motor nerve

All the systems concerned in the control of movement—the corticospinal pathway, descending extrapyramidal fibres, spinal interneurones and proprioceptive afferents—converge on the lower motor neurone. The cell bodies of these neurones are found in the anterior horn of spinal grey matter and they are sometimes known as *anterior horn cells*. The axons of these cells form the final common pathway for neural activation of muscle contraction.

Lower motor neurones do more than convey impulses to the neuromuscular junction. They also exert a trophic influence on the muscle fibres that they innervate. If the neurone is destroyed the specialized area of the muscle cell membrane which forms the neuromuscular junction degenerates and the whole of the surface of the muscle fibre becomes sensitive to acetyl choline. Production of cholin esterase, the enzyme which inactivates acetyl choline, by the postsynaptic membrane is reduced. Denervated muscle fibres may become reinnervated by branches from other lower motor neurones but, if this process fails, the muscle fibre eventually atrophies.

Denervated muscle fibres show spontaneous activity perhaps partly because of their supersensitivity to acetyl choline. This activity can be detected by a needle electrode inserted into the muscle or seen as twitches or ripples of the skin overlying the muscle. Visible spontaneous contractions are known as *fasciculations* and represent activity in a whole motor unit (i.e. all the muscle fibres innervated by a single motor neurone). Contractions of a single muscle fibre are known as *fibrillations* and can only be detected electrically.

CLINICAL EXAMINATION OF THE MOTOR SYSTEM

There are five parts to the examination of the motor system:

1. Observation of the patient
2. Assessment of muscle tone
3. Assessment of muscle power

4. Tests of co-ordination
5. Examination of reflexes.

Observation of the patient

Information that you have obtained while taking the history may suggest particular features to look out for. Otherwise try to ask yourself some of the following questions.

Muscle

Are there any signs of muscle wasting? Look both at the proximal musculature of the shoulder and hip girdles and distally at the small muscles of the hands and the calves and feet. Are there any deformities present which might indicate long-standing muscle imbalance? Clawing of the hand and pes cavus are examples; these deformities are the result of weakness of the intrinsic muscles of the hand and foot respectively.

Look for fasciculations. These are a sign of denervation of muscle and usually indicate disease affecting anterior horn cells.

Limbs

Is there any asymmetry of limb length or development? A long-standing neurological lesion, especially if it has been present since childhood, often results in poorer development of the affected limb.

Involuntary movements

Are any involuntary movements present? Which part of the body is affected? Are the movements stereotyped or is the pattern different each time? Try to categorize the movements into tremor, chorea, athetosis, or hemiballismus.

Bradykinesia

Observe if the patient has any difficulty with the initiation of movements. Does his face lack animation and expression?

Gait

If possible, watch the patient walking at a time when he is unaware of your gaze. Observe the posture of his body, the regularity and length of his stride, how easily he stops, starts and turns around, whether he swings his arms and if he can maintain steady balance and a straight course. Some characteristic abnormalities of gait are shown in Figure 2.7.

Muscle tone

Most medical students and many doctors neglect to test muscle tone or, if they do test it, perform the examination so badly that they obtain no useful information. This is a pity because alteration in muscle tone is a valuable physical sign in disease of both corticospinal and extrapyramidal systems.

What is meant by muscle tone? For clinical purposes, muscle tone means the tension in *resting* muscle. In practice you assess tone by gauging the resistance felt as you put the patient's joint through a full range of passive movement.

The patient needs to be able to relax completely so the examination must be performed with him lying on a bed or couch. Reassure the patient that you won't hurt him and make sure that you keep your word. Remember that joint disease is common and be particularly careful with elderly patients. Arthritis will, of course, tend to increase the feeling of resistance to passive movement of the joint even when resting muscle tone is normal.

To examine tone in the upper limbs start by putting wrist and elbow joints through the full range of extension and flexion. Then grasp the patient's hand as if you were going to shake hands with him and pronate and supinate his forearm. Carry out these movements slowly at first and then more rapidly.

Test muscle tone in the lower limbs by flexing and extending the knee. It often helps to start by rolling the extended leg with your hand on the patient's shin to produce alternate internal and external rotation of the leg. This allows you to assess tone in the hip girdle muscles. It also encourages the patient to relax and you can take the opportunity to observe how the foot flops from side to side with the muscles which control the ankle joint relaxed.

All techniques of physical examination get easier with practice. Partly this is just a matter of acquiring facility in doing the test but, especially where the assessment of tone is concerned, repeated practice allows you to build up experience of the range of what

L. Hemiplegia. The arm is held in a flexed position. Flexion of the leg is weak so it is brought forward by circumduction. The patient wears out the toe of his shoe

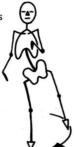

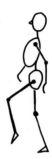

Footdrop. Because dorsiflexion is weak at the ankle, he must walk with a high-stepping gait to avoid tripping.

Spastic paraparesis. Both legs are weak and spastic. Increased tone in the adductors leads to a scissors gait. The patient tends to walk upon his toes

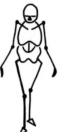

Ataxia. The patient walks with a broad-based gait, reeling about and swinging his arms in an attempt to maintain balance

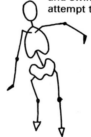

Parkinsonism. The patient stands in a flexed posture. Arms are held at waist level. He walks with short, shuffling steps

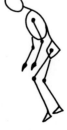

Fig. 2.7   Abnormalities of gait.

is normal. For both reasons it is worth examining muscle tone in patients who have no neurological disease.

There are two patterns of increased muscle tone: spasticity and rigidity:

Spasticity

As you attempt to put the joint through its range of movement, the initial resistance is high and then it suddenly subsides. The sensation is often described as being like closing a clasp-knife. This type of increase in muscle tone is known as spasticity.

Spasticity is found when a lesion of the corticospinal tract is present. It tends to be most evident in the antigravity muscles and it can usually be detected most clearly in the quadriceps muscle when attempting to flex the patient's knee rapidly from a fully extended position.

When spasticity is present, *clonus* can often be elicited. Clonus is a repetitive rhythmic series of involuntary muscle contractions produced in response to a sudden stretch of the muscle. Figure 2.8 illustrates the method of producing patellar clonus by suddenly stretching the quadriceps with a sharp push of the patella towards the foot, and ankle clonus by a sudden dorsiflexion of the

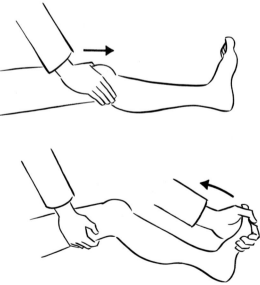

Fig. 2.8 How to elicit patellar and ankle clonus.

foot to give a sharp stretch to the calf muscles. Deliver the stretch briskly and maintain the pressure.

A few beats of clonus are quite commonly elicited in normal individuals but, if sustained, clonus is strong evidence of a cortico-spinal tract lesion. Occasionally, sustained clonus is found in normal but very apprehensive people. Those of you who go rock climbing may have observed it in yourselves when, scared half to death in an exposed and precarious position, your foot jumps up and down uncontrollably as you step up on to a small toe hold.

Rigidity

Increased muscle tone felt throughout the whole range of movement of a joint is known as rigidity. It is usually described as being like bending a lead pipe and is characteristic of lesions in the extra-pyramidal system. Tremor is often found in extrapyramidal disease and may be superimposed on rigidity. This gives a rather jerky feel as the joint is flexed and extended—a phenomenon referred to as *cogwheel* rigidity. Rigidity of the cogwheel type may sometimes be found in patients who do not have a visible tremor at rest.

Decreased muscle tone

In the normal relaxed person muscle tone is very low which, of course, makes it very difficult to appreciate when *hypotonia* is present. Don't worry too much about detecting reduction in muscle tone. Honest physicians will admit that it is something of a make-weight sign, looked for only when a diagnosis of a disease known to produce hypotonia has already been established from the presence of other, more reliable, clinical signs.

When you examine muscle tone concentrate on trying to detect increased tone and deciding whether the pattern of the increase in tone is spasticity or rigidity.

Muscle power

The chain of events leading to a voluntarily initiated full-strength muscle contraction has a number of links, all of which must be intact if the muscle is to develop its full power. The most important of these links are shown in Figure 2.9.

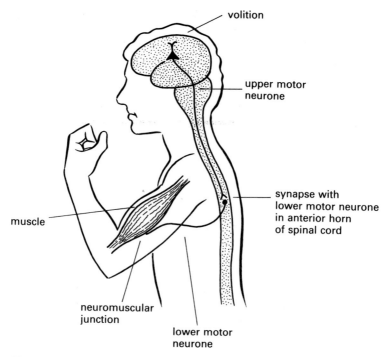

Fig. 2.9 The pathway for voluntary muscle contraction.

It is obvious that the patient must be prepared to make a full effort to contract the muscle or an apparent weakness will be found. Patients often need quite vigorous encouragement to do this. Bear in mind that from the patient's point of view, what you are asking him to do may seem a little odd. You must ensure that he understands clearly what is required. Although a request such as 'flex your fingers' or 'pronate your forearm' may be straightforward enough to a medical student who has studied anatomy for three terms, it is likely to mystify most patients.

It is quite impossible and entirely unnecessary to test the power of every muscle in the body. For most purposes the short routine shown in Figure 2.10 will be satisfactory. The basic principle is to get the patient to produce a full strength contraction of a muscle group against resistance provided by you, the examiner. In this way you can assess the muscle power of the patient by comparing his strength with your own. Be at some pains to avoid giving a display of your own machismo and be absolutely certain not to hurt the patient.

Degrees of muscle weakness are graded according to the following scale:

5 Full strength muscle contraction
4 Reduced strength contraction but active movement possible against gravity and resistance
3 Movement possible against gravity only
2 Movement possible only if the effect of gravity is eliminated
1 Flicker of contraction seen in the muscle but no movement
0 No contraction visible.

The detection of muscle weakness indicates dysfunction at one of the levels in the pathway shown in Figure 2.9. It does not, by itself, indicate where the lesion lies. However, lesions at particular levels tend to produce characteristic patterns of weakness and recognition of these patterns is often an important clue to diagnosis.

Weakness caused by lesions in the corticospinal pathways

There is poor performance of rapid repetitive fine finger movements. Weakness is most evident in the extensor muscle groups of the upper limb (deltoid, triceps, wrist and finger extensors) and in the flexor muscles of the lower limb (iliopsoas, hamstrings, peronei and tibialis anterior). This pattern is known as a *pyramidally distributed weakness*.

Proximal weakness

Symmetrical weakness confined mainly to the muscles of the shoulder and hip girdles suggests primary muscle disease or a myopathy secondary to systemic disease.

Distal weakness

Weakness confined to the distal extremities of limbs is often the result of peripheral nerve disease. One form of muscular dystrophy, dystrophia myotonica, is unusual in affecting distal muscles more severely than proximal muscles.

Fluctuating weakness

Muscle weakness that varies in severity over a short space of time,

Shoulder abduction
muscle: deltoid
peripheral nerve: axillary
roots: C5, 6

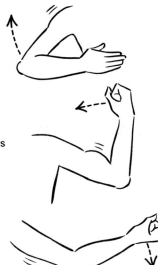

Elbow flexion
muscle: biceps
peripheral nerve: musculocutaneous
roots: C5, 6

Elbow extension
muscle: triceps
peripheral nerve: radial
roots: C7, 8

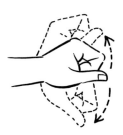

Wrist extension
muscles: extensor carpi radialis
          extensor carpi ulnaris
peripheral nerves: radial
roots: C6, 7, 8

Wrist flexion
muscles: flexor carpi radialis
          flexor carpi ulnaris
peripheral nerves: ulnar
                    median
roots: C6, 7, 8, T1

Finger extension
muscle: extensor digitorum
peripheral nerve; radial
roots: C7, 8

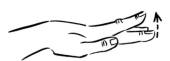

Finger abduction
muscles: abductor digiti minimi
          dorsal interossei
peripheral nerve: ulnar
roots: C8, T1

Thumb abduction
muscle: abductor pollicis brevis
peripheral nerve: median
roots: C8, T1

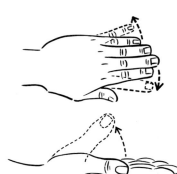

Hip flexion
muscle: iliopsoas
peripheral nerves: spinal
branches of L1, 2
roots: L1, 2

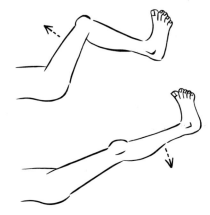

Hip extension
muscle: gluteus maximus
peripheral nerve: inferior gluteal
roots: L5, S1

Knee extension
muscle: quadriceps
peripheral nerve: femoral
roots: L2, 3, 4

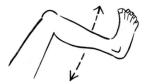

Knee flexion
muscle: hamstrings
peripheral nerve: sciatic
roots: L5, S1, 2

Dorsiflexion of foot
muscle: tibialis anterior
peripheral nerve: deep peroneal
roots: L4, 5

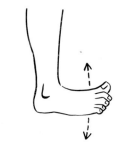

Plantar flexion of foot
muscles: gastrocnemius
         soleus
peripheral nerve: deep peroneal
roots: S1, 2

Inversion of foot
muscle: tibialis posterior
peripheral nerve: posterior tibial
roots: L4, 5

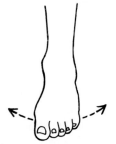

Eversion of foot
muscles: peroneii
peripheral nerve: superficial peroneal
roots: L5, S1

Fig. 2.10   The examination of muscle strength.

especially if it can be influenced by vigorous encouragement from the examiner, may be an indication that the patient's complaints are functional rather than organic in origin.

Fatiguability

An exaggeration of the normal phenomenon of muscle fatigue with exercise is typical of myasthenia gravis. The patient complains of weakness that is worse after exercise or at the end of the day.

Localized weakness

Weakness localized to one particular muscle or muscle group is frequently the result of a localized lesion in the distal part of the pathway shown in Figure 2.9, often in a nerve root or a peripheral nerve. This straightforward interpretation should be treated with circumspection because small localized lesions anywhere in the motor pathway from the motor cortex to the muscle itself can produce relatively isolated muscle weakness.

Co-ordination

The ability to co-ordinate muscular movement requires both intact cerebellar function and normal proprioception. If either of these systems is malfunctioning the patient will exhibit ataxia.

Inco-ordination of the muscles of the axial skeleton gives rise to *truncal ataxia*. It can be detected by observing the patient's gait; he is unsteady even standing still and finds it difficult or impossible to walk along a straight line. Most medical students will have had first hand experience of the temporary depression of normal cerebellar function produced by ethanol. Patients with truncal ataxia often spontaneously describe their gait as being as if they were drunk. Asking the patient to walk heel to toe may reveal more minor degrees of truncal ataxia.

Examine co-ordination of the upper limbs by the finger–nose test. Ask the patient first to put his index finger on the tip of his nose and then to reach out and touch your finger held a couple of feet away. He should then move his finger to and fro between the tip of his nose and the tip of your finger. Figure 2.11 makes the procedure clear. When disease of the cerebellum is present the patient misjudges the effort required to make the movement and tends to overshoot the target. This phenomenon is known as

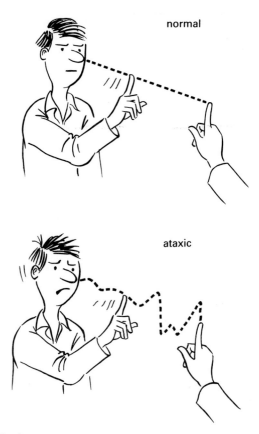

normal

ataxic

Fig. 2.11   The finger–nose test.

past-pointing. Instead of the muscles of the shoulder, elbow and wrist operating smoothly together the movement is broken up into its constituent parts and becomes jerky. As the finger approaches its target minor errors of direction are grossly overcorrected and an *intention tremor* becomes apparent.

The heel–shin test is used to detect ataxia of the lower limbs. The patient is asked to place the heel of his right foot on his left knee and then to slide the right heel up and down the full length of his shin. The test must then be repeated with the patient using his other leg. He should be able to maintain his heel on the anterior edge of his opposite tibia throughout the movement.

Ataxia can be caused either by proprioceptive sensory loss or by cerebellar dysfunction. The most reliable way to distinguish between these two causes is to carry out an independent test of proprioceptive function and a technique for doing this will be described in Chapter 3. However, it is sometimes possible to discriminate between the two types of ataxia by asking the patient to perform the finger–nose and heel–shin tests with his eyes closed. Visual information can, to some extent, compensate for diminished proprioceptive input. If the ataxia becomes much worse when the patient closes his eyes it is likely to be caused by dysfunction in the sensory pathways to the cerebellum rather than by a lesion in the cerebellum itself.

Examination of reflexes

Tendon reflexes

Reread the section on the anatomy of the muscle stretch reflex (pages 18–20) to be sure that you understand that when you hit a tendon with your hammer and observe the resulting muscle contraction you are testing:

1. that the sensory fibres of the peripheral nerve will conduct a volley of afferent proprioceptive impulses
2. the integrity of synaptic transmission between the sensory and the motor neurones in the spinal cord, and the level of excitability of the motor neurone pool
3. the function of the lower motor neurone pathway from the anterior horn of spinal cord grey matter to the neuromuscular junction.

If a tendon reflex is present you can deduce that all three parts of the reflex are functioning. Pathologically brisk reflexes indicate that the descending inhibitory influences on the motor neurone pool are reduced and therefore that a structural lesion in the corticospinal tract is probably present. An absent reflex indicates dysfunction in one or more of the three parts of the reflex pathway but does not, by itself, localize the lesion.

In order to be able to interpret an abnormality in a tendon reflex you need to know which segmental level of the spinal cord and which peripheral nerve mediates that particular reflex. This information, together with the method of eliciting the tendon reflexes is shown in Figure 2.12.

Bear in mind the following few points concerning technique and interpretation. It is much easier to elicit a tendon reflex if the patient is relaxed. Getting a patient to relax during a physical examination can be very difficult, especially if he is anxious.

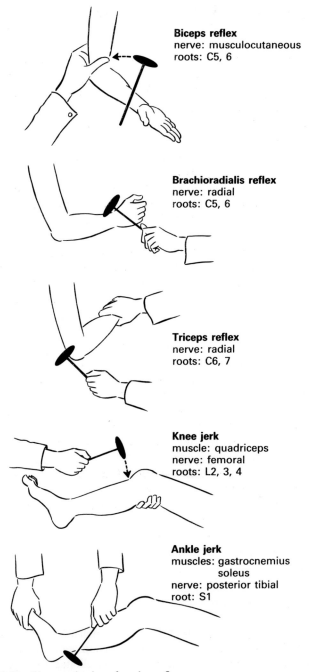

Biceps reflex
nerve: musculocutaneous
roots: C5, 6

Brachioradialis reflex
nerve: radial
roots: C5, 6

Triceps reflex
nerve: radial
roots: C6, 7

Knee jerk
muscle: quadriceps
nerve: femoral
roots: L2, 3, 4

Ankle jerk
muscles: gastrocnemius
                soleus
nerve: posterior tibial
root: S1

Fig. 2.12   The examination of tendon reflexes.

Try paraphrasing the simple command 'relax'; for example, 'let yourself go loose'. Don't be in a hurry and never get irritated by a patient's failure to relax. Losing your temper is a futile way of trying to induce a state of muscular relaxation in a patient. Make sure that you hit the tendon in the right place. This is especially important with the triceps jerk, because the tendon is very short, and with the knee jerk, because the joint is so often deformed by arthritis and it is easy to hit the head of the tibia instead of the patellar tendon.

When eliciting the brachioradialis reflex the technique is to put your left thumb over the insertion of the muscle into the radius and to hit your own thumb with the tendon hammer. Although this does not stretch the muscle directly, the vibration induced by the blow from the hammer stimulates the stretch receptors within the muscle.

Compare the tendon reflexes of one side of the body with those of the opposite side. First test the left biceps jerk then compare it with the right. Then do the same with the left and right brachioradialis jerks, and so on. Normally, tendon reflexes are symmetrical in their amplitude and asymmetry is an early clue that a lesion of the corticospinal tract is present.

Never conclude that a reflex is absent until you have tried reinforcing it. To reinforce upper limb reflexes ask the patient to clench his teeth or to make a tight fist with the opposite hand. He should do this just as you strike the tendon and relax immediately afterwards. The lower limb reflexes can be reinforced by Jendrassik's manoeuvre. The patient hooks the flexed fingers of his two hands together and pulls hard. Again he should make the effort just before you hit the tendon.

The decision as to whether the reflexes are pathologically brisk or not may be difficult. Asymmetry of reflexes usually indicates disease but if all the tendon reflexes are symmetrically brisk you should be chary of diagnosing corticospinal tract lesions unless there is corroborative evidence from the superficial reflexes. The apparent hyper-reflexia may only be a reflection of the patient's anxiety.

Superficial reflexes

There are only two superficial reflexes of importance: the *plantar reflex* and the *abdominal reflexes*. Unlike tendon reflexes these are polysynaptic and nociceptive—that is to say, elicited by a painful

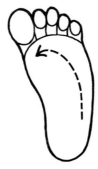

Fig. 2.13   How to elicit the plantar reflex.

stimulus. The neurophysiology of the plantar reflex is complicated and controversial. Take a pragmatic view and accept that
the normal plantar response is flexion of the big toe at the meta-
tarsal-phalangeal joint. Extension of the toe at the same joint is
abnormal and is a reliable indicator of a lesion in the corticospinal
tract. The technique of eliciting a plantar reflex is shown in Figure
2.13. Use the end of a tendon hammer, an orange stick or a key.
Avoid stimulating the flexor surfaces of the toes. Start the stroke
with light pressure and gradually increase the intensity of the
stimulus until a response is elicited. If you ask a colleague to test
your own plantar reflexes you will be able to appreciate why most
patients find this test unpleasant. You should always warn the
patient that you are about to perform this test and request him to
try not to jerk his foot away.

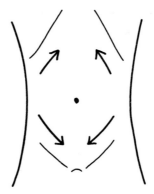

Fig 2.14   The abdominal reflexes.

Abdominal reflexes can be elicited from most normal people. They are generally lost in disease of the corticospinal tracts but absence of these reflexes is a rather less reliable indication of this than an extensor plantar response. It may be difficult or impossible to elicit the abdominal reflexes in patients who are very obese, multiparous or who have undergone several laparotomies. Use an orange stick or some other moderately pointed but noncutting device. Stroke the skin of the anterior abdominal wall with a brisk medially directed movement in each of the four quadrants. Look for a brief contraction of the underlying muscle and deviation of the umbilicus towards the stimulated quadrant (see Fig. 2.14).

Table 2.1 Summary of the examination of the motor system

Observation	Muscle wasting and fasciculation
	Involuntary movements
	Bradykinesia
	Gait
Muscle tone	Rigidity
	Spasticity
Muscle power	Systematic testing of power in upper and lower limbs
Co-ordination	Finger–nose test
	Heel–shin test
Tendon reflexes	Biceps
	Triceps
	Brachioradialis
	Knee
	Ankle
Superficial reflexes	Plantar reflex
	Abdominal reflexes

3. The sensory system

NEUROANATOMY AND NEUROPHYSIOLOGY

Although, strictly speaking, the term sensory system includes the special senses and visceral sensation, this chapter is concerned only with somatic sensation. Somatic sensation consists of exteroceptive sensory information obtained from free nerve endings and receptors located superficially and proprioceptive sensation, concerned with body position and movement, gained from stretch receptors in muscle, tendons, ligaments and joint capsules.

Peripheral receptors and sensory modalities

There has been a long argument about whether peripheral nerve endings are specific to particular sensory modalities or whether our sensory perception depends only upon the spatial and temporal pattern of stimulation of nerve endings. Some physiologists have suggested that the different types of structures seen at the nerve terminals in histological preparations of skin are no more than artefact; others have asserted that they are specialized receptors which transduce certain forms of energy with particular efficiency and endow the nerve ending with specificity. Some sensory nerve endings in the skin must be more responsive to one type of stimulus than another and to that extent, at least, nerve endings are modality specific. If all endings were equally likely to respond no matter what the nature of the stimulus, there would be no way in which we could discriminate one type of stimulus from another. In fact we are very good at distinguishing a wide range of cutaneous sensations—heat, cold, smoothness, roughness, wetness, dryness, sliminess, hardness, softness and many others. There is no need to postulate say, a specialized nerve ending for the sensation of sliminess but, obviously, the patterns of response in cutaneous nerve endings when we touch a greasy formica table-top cannot be the same as those produced when we touch the dry abrasive surface of a sheet of sandpaper.

Neurologists and physiologists tend to concentrate on the modalities of temperature, touch, vibration and pain. These modalities are correlated anatomically with hot and cold receptors, slowly adapting mechanoreceptors, rapidly adapting mechanoreceptors and nociceptive free nerve endings. There is some physiological justification for considering these modalities primary and for thinking that other cutaneous sensations are derived from different combinations of these modalities. The analogy here is with artists who can mix a whole palate of hues from three primary colours. A child with a paint-box, however, sees no reason why his pink or mauve tints are any less primary than his reds or blues and you will find that most patients with sensory disturbance describe their symptoms in terms other than these primary sensory modalities.

Sensory nerve endings are not evenly distributed over the body surface. A moment's introspection will remind you that the hands and face, especially the finger tips and the lips, are able to provide a much richer tactile experience than the elbow or the buttock.

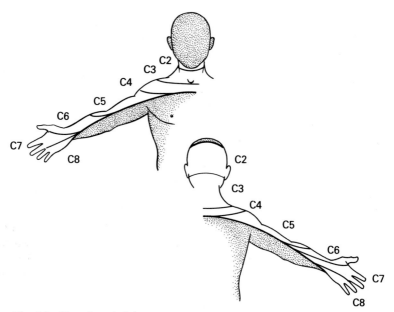

Fig. 3.1 Map of cervical dermatomes.

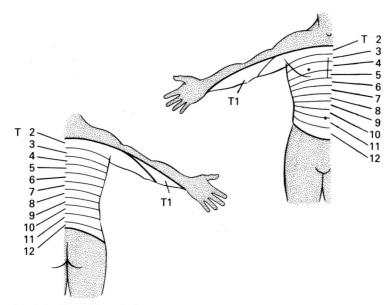

Fig. 3.2   Map of thoracic dermatomes.

The former areas are, of course, much more plentifully supplied with sensory nerves than the latter and the amount of sensory cortex in the brain which corresponds to lips and finger tips is disproportionately large. If, when examining a patient's sensory system, you apply a stimulus to his finger he should be able to localize it precisely and distinguish the type of sensation. But do not expect the same accuracy of response if you apply the same stimulus to his trunk or to his leg.

Peripheral sensory nerves

Information about noxious and painful stimuli and temperature is carried by small diameter non-myelinated or thinly myelinated nerve fibres. Larger diameter myelinated fibres are reserved for information about touch and vibration and the largest fibres of all transmit proprioceptive information from muscle spindles, tendon organs and joint position receptors. All sensory fibres enter the spinal cord by the dorsal (posterior) root and have their cell bodies located just outside the spinal cord in the dorsal root ganglion. The cutaneous area supplied by the sensory nerve fibres entering the spinal cord through one dorsal root corresponds to

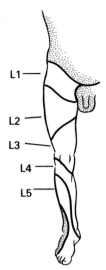

Fig. 3.3 Map of lumbar dermatomes.

the dermatome of that root. Dermatomes are fairly constant topographically from individual to individual (see Figs 3.1 to 3.4 for maps of dermatomes) and sensory disturbance restricted to a dermatomal distribution is characteristic of a lesion affecting the

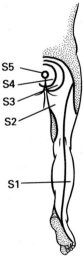

Fig. 3.4 Map of sacral dermatomes.

nerve root. However, there is considerable overlap between dermatomes so that a lesion restricted to one sensory root does not usually cause much sensory loss.

Central sensory pathways

There are two major anatomical pathways involved with conscious sensation: the dorsal column—lemniscal system and the spinothalamic pathways.

Dorsal column—lemniscal system

Large diameter axons serving the modalities of touch and proprioception predominate. The pathway is uncrossed in the spinal cord and ascends ipsilaterally in the dorsal columns to the gracile and cuneate nuclei in the lower medulla. Second order neurones arising from these nuclei decussate within the medulla to form the medial lemniscus. The fibres of the medial lemniscus travel to the ventroposterolateral nuclei of the thalamus and, from there, third order fibres project to the primary somatosensory cortex in the parietal lobe. Accurate point-to-point mapping is preserved throughout—an arrangement which is in keeping with the known function of this pathway in tactile discrimination and localization. The important anatomical features of the pathway are shown in Figure 3.5. The integrity of the dorsal column lemniscal system is tested by using a piece of cotton-wool to examine the modality of fine touch, a tuning fork to examine transmission from the rapidly adapting touch receptors and by moving a small joint to examine conscious proprioceptive sensation.

Spinothalamic system

The spinothalamic pathways consist of smaller diameter nerve fibres carrying the modalities of pain and temperature. Touch is also carried in this pathway but information about spatial localization is less precise than in the dorsal columns. Unlike the fibres carried in the dorsal columns the peripheral nerve fibres of the spinothalamic system synapse in the grey matter of the dorsal horn of the spinal cord at or just above the level at which they enter the cord. Second order fibres decussate immediately in the anterior commissure of the cord. They then travel rostrally in the spinothalamic tracts. Numerous collateral fibres are given off to

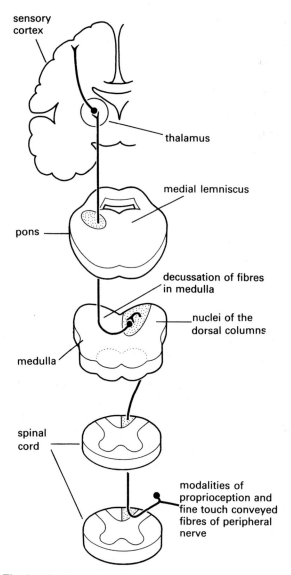

Fig. 3.5 The dorsal column—lemniscal system.

the reticular formation as the pathway ascends. In the medulla the tract lies just lateral to the medial lemniscus and travels alongside it to the posterior nuclei of the thalamus. From here fibres are distributed to the sensory cortex. Figure 3.6 shows this pathway.

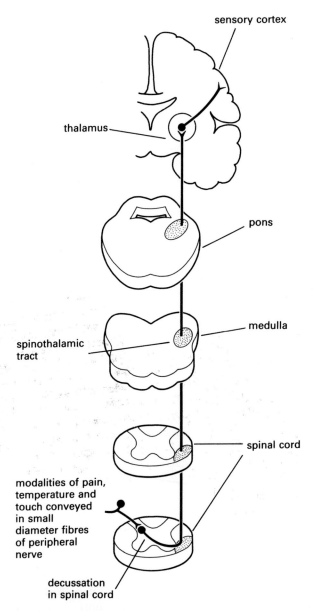

Fig. 3.6   The spinothalamic system.

Clinical examination of the spinothalamic system involves testing the patient's perception of pain and temperature.

The sensory information transmitted in the spinothalamic tracts carries a large affective component. This is perhaps not surprising since the transmission of pain is a major function of the spinothalamic system. In some ways pain is better thought of as an emotional state than as a sensory modality. It is a matter of everyday experience that one's perception of a painful stimulus is very dependent on the circumstances under which it was sustained. A kick on the shins which would have one yelling with pain if it occurred while one was waiting for a bus is scarcely noticed during a game of hockey. There are many extreme examples of this phenomenon from soldiers who sustained severe injuries on the battlefield but who felt no pain for many hours afterwards.

The traffic of painful impulses ascending in the spinothalamic tracts is strongly influenced by simultaneous afferent sensory information entering the spinal cord through large diameter fibres destined to travel in the dorsal columns. Collaterals from these large axons enter the grey matter of the dorsal horn and by inhibition of relay cells may modify the transmission of nerve impulses in the smaller diameter spinothalamic fibres. This is a very simplified version of the gate control theory of the modulation of transmission of impulses from nociceptive afferents by other afferent impulses. An everyday example of gate control is the way in which a painful spot can be eased by rubbing hard on the area of skin around it. Transmission of pain in the spinothalamic tracts is also modified by descending fibres from three supraspinal areas: the periaqueductal grey matter in the mid-brain, the locus ceruleus in the pons and the raphe nuclei in the medulla. It is interesting that one of these areas, the periaqueductal grey matter, is known to contain opiate receptors.

Table 3.1 summarizes the important features of the dorsal column lemniscal system and spinothalamic system.

The thalamus

The thalamus is the major sensory relay for both dorsal column and spinothalamic systems and massive fibre projections travel from it to the cortical sensory areas in the parietal lobes. Lesions within the thalamus cause impairment of somatic sensation, hypoaesthesia, often affecting the whole of the contralateral half of the body. A peculiar feature is that the sensory loss may be ac-

Table 3.1 Pathways of conscious sensation

Modality	Fibre type	Pathway	Function
Dorsal column—leminiscal system			
Touch Proprioception Vibration	Large, myelinated	Ipsilateral in spinal cord, decussates in the medulla to form the medial leminiscus	Carries information about type and precise localization of the stimulus
Spinothalamic system			
Pain Temperature Touch	Small, unmyelinated and thinly myelinated fibres	Fibres decussate within a short distance of entering spinal cord and then ascend in the contralateral spinothalamic tract	Important affective component to sensory information

companied by spontaneous pain in the absence of any peripheral stimulation. In addition, innocuous low-intensity stimuli—for example, a light touch—may be perceived as an unpleasant tingling or burning sensation. This phenomenon is known as *dysaesthesia*.

The sensory cortex

Cutaneous sensation is not a passive process. Think how much easier it is to form an impression of the texture of a surface if you run your fingers over it rather than just lay your hand on it. The analysis of sensory information takes place in the parietal cortex and the close anatomical relationship to the motor cortex lying just anteriorly is unlikely to be accidental. Presumably, decoding and processing of afferent sensory information in the sensory cortex is most efficient if there is a parallel input of motor information.

Lesions in the sensory cortical areas show themselves not by producing cutaneous anaesthesia but by a reduction in ability to discriminate between and find meaning in sensory stimuli. The patient's appreciation of a simple stimulus like a pin-prick may remain relatively unimpaired, but if you ask him to put his hand in his pocket and take out a coin he may well extract his key-ring instead.

EXAMINATION OF SENSATION

All parts of the clinical examination start with observation and examination of sensation is no exception. Denervated skin heals less quickly than normal and is more susceptible to damage. Look for evidence that an area of the body is anaesthetic or hypoaesthetic; a cigarette smoker may burn his fingers if he has lost awareness of pain and temperature, ulcers can occur on the feet of patients with severe polyneuropathy and a joint can become distorted and disorganized (a Charcot joint) if pain sensation is no longer present to warn of excessive forces being applied.

Now test the modalities of pain, light touch, joint position and vibration. Temperature perception is not usually tested as a routine, but you need to know how to do it and to be aware of the circumstances when it may provide useful information. Finally, test the function of the sensory cortex.

The examination of sensation requires the active co-operation of the patient to be successful. If you try to be too meticulous you run the risk of the patient becoming bored and losing his concentration. If you perform the examination too rapidly you may miss a significant sensory deficit. When the patient's history has led you to expect a sensory loss start the examination in the area most likely to be affected. If there are no clues from the history it is usually best to start the examination in the distal part of the limbs and move proximally.

Pain

Use a hat pin or an ordinary dress-maker's pin, but never a hypodermic needle, to test pain sensation. The latter is so sharp that it penetrates the skin too easily and painlessly. The safe way to hold the pin is with the shaft between your index finger and thumb. It is then almost impossible to grip it tightly enough to be able to penetrate the patient's skin. Remember to warn the patient of what you are about to do; an unexpected stab with a pin won't help you to gain his co-operation. Ask him if he feels the sharp pricking sensation normally. Everyone has pricked themselves with a pin at some time so your patient will know the quality of the sensation that he should experience. Start the examination distally in the legs and arms and move proximally. If the patient's perception of pin prick is reduced in the extremities of the limbs it may be helpful to ask him to indicate the point at which the sensation becomes sharper as you move the stimulus proximally.

Remember that the finger tips, which are very sensitive to touch, are relatively insensitive to pain. Delineate any area of reduced or absent sensation carefully and try to determine if it corresponds to the distribution of a peripheral nerve or dermatome.

Light touch

A small piece of cotton wool provides the best stimulus for testing tactile sensation. Follow the same plan of testing as for pain.

Joint position

Test joint position sensation at the distal interphalangeal joints of the hallux and index finger. Immobilize the proximal joints with one hand and, holding it between your thumb and forefinger, move the terminal phalanx a few degrees up or down. Explain clearly to the patient that you want him to report the direction of movement.

Vibration

A 128 cycles per second tuning fork is applied to the dorsum of the hallux. It is essential that the patient understands that he is being asked to report the sensation of vibration and not merely the feeling of pressure from the base of the tuning fork. If he can feel vibration on the hallux there is no need to test more proximally but if vibration sensation is absent there, repeat the test on the medial malleolus, tibial tuberosity, iliac crests, costal margins and sternum until you find the level at which vibration is first felt.

Temperature

The cold metal of the end of your tendon hammer or of the tines of the tuning fork usually provides an adequate stimulus to test perception of cold. It is more trouble but more satisfactory to fill two identical small blood specimen tubes, one with warm and one with cold water, to check if the patient can distinguish between them.

Tests of cortical sensation

Tests of cortical sensation are only useful if the simple tests just described show peripheral sensation to be intact. *Stereognosis* refers to the ability to identify an object placed in the hand without look-ing at it. By tradition, neurologists carry a champagne cork in their pocket as the test object. This scores high marks for panache, but since the object is outside the cultural experience of many patients (and beyond the purse of most medical students) it is better to sub-stitute a more everyday item such as a pen or a coin. *Graphaes-thesia* is the ability to identify a letter or a digit inscribed on the palm of the hand. Use a pencil to avoid marking the patient. An alternative is to use a pair of dividers with blunt tips or an un-wound paperclip to test *two-point discrimination*. Randomly apply stimuli of one point or two to the finger tip of the patient. Start with the points about 10 mm apart and gradually move the points closer until the patient is unable to tell whether you have touched him with one point or two. Subjects with normal sensation can distinguish two points as close as 3 or 4 mm on a finger tip.

4. The cranial nerves

Testing the function of the cranial nerves should be part of the physical examination carried out on every patient. This chapter outlines the essential anatomy and physiology that you need to know in order to perform the examination intelligently and describes the method of examination of each of the cranial nerves.

THE OLFACTORY (I) NERVES

These very short nerves carry information about smell from receptors in the olfactory mucosa of the nasopharynx through the cribriform plate in the base of the anterior cranial fossa to the olfactory bulbs. Second order neurones arising in the bulbs travel in the olfactory tracts to the medial part of the cortex of the temporal lobes.

Examination

Smell is tested in each nostril individually. Occlude one of the patient's nostrils with a finger and, using something aromatic but not too pungent from the bedside locker (an orange or a bar of scented soap will serve admirably), ask him if he can smell it. A collection of smell bottles each containing an arcane odoriferous substance can usually be found at the back of a dusty cupboard in a neurological ward—tacit testimony to the unreliability of clinical examination of this pathway. Loss of sense of smell is more often due to local disease of the olfactory mucosa rather than a neurological lesion.

THE OPTIC (II) NERVES

The examination of the optic pathways includes the measurement of visual acuity, the testing of visual fields and observation of the head of the optic nerve with an ophthalmoscope. The pupillary reflexes depend on the integrity of both the optic and oculomotor nerves and are discussed in the next section.

Visual acuity

Visual acuity is a test of macular vision. Although the macula forms only a small part of the retina it gives rise to the majority of fibres in the optic nerve. Lesions of the optic nerve cause a profound deterioration in visual acuity.

Examination

Acuity is best tested using a Snellen chart at a distance of 6 metres but a card printed with standard test type of different sizes is an adequate substitute for the bed-bound patient. Test each eye individually and allow the patient to wear his spectacles.

Visual fields

The most important features of the visual pathways are illustrated in very simple form in Figure 4.1. It is crucial to understand the anatomy to be able to interpret visual field defects. An object in the left half of the visual field is seen by the nasal half of the retina of the left eye and the temporal half of the retina of the right eye. Because of the partial decussation of the optic nerves at the *optic chiasm* all the nerve fibres from these parts of the retinae project to the right occipital cortex. Similarly, encoded images of objects on the right side get sent to the visual cortex of the left hemisphere. This arrangement, of course, parallels that of the motor and sensory systems. Lesions in the frontal or parietal lobes of one cerebral hemisphere cause a contralateral hemiparesis or a contralateral hemianaesthesia; it is not surprising that a lesion in the occipital lobe should cause a contralateral hemianopia.

The nomenclature of field defects sometimes causes confusion. The visual fields are always referred to from the patient's point of view. A patient with a left homonymous hemianopia for example, cannot see to the left out of either eye.

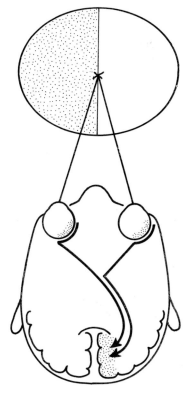

Fig. 4.1   The visual pathway. The left visual field projects to the right hemisphere.

Patterns of visual field loss

A lesion in an optic nerve causes a field defect in one eye only. As noted above, this defect is likely to affect macular vision and cause a serious loss of visual acuity.

A lesion at the optic chiasm usually results in a bitemporal hemianopia. This is because the majority of chiasmal lesions are the result of upward expansion of pituitary tumours. The central part of the chiasm is compressed and it is this part that carries the decussating fibres from the nasal halves, and therefore the temporal fields, of both retinae. Very rarely, an expanding pituitary tumour causes bilateral nasal field defects by encircling the chiasm and compressing it from a lateral direction.

Lesions behind the optic chiasm cause homonymous defects of

one half of the visual field. This is true whether the lesion is situated in the optic tract, the optic radiation or in the visual cortex.

The visual fields depend on normal retinal function as well as intact visual pathways. Concentric restriction of visual fields can result from retinal degeneration and glaucoma.

Examination

Test the visual fields of your patient by comparing them with your own. The technique is long-winded to describe but quick to perform. It is illustrated in Figure 4.2. Position yourself face to face with the patient about a metre away. To test the visual field of the patient's left eye, ask him to cover his right eye with his hand and occlude your own left eye. Instruct him to look directly into your open eye; apart from ensuring that your visual fields match, this allows you to be sure that he maintains fixation. Bring your pointed index finger or the head of a hat pin towards the centre of the visual field from beyond the periphery of vision and tell him to report when he is first aware of seeing it. Both you and the patient should register the stimulus at the same time. It is important to bring in the stimulus fairly slowly so that he has time to respond. Because most visual field defects split the visual field along the vertical meridian it is necessary to bring in the stimulus

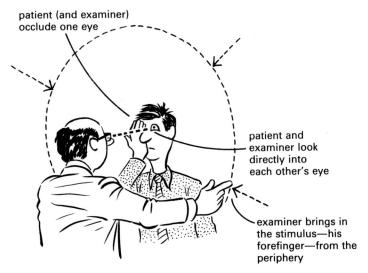

patient (and examiner) occlude one eye

patient and examiner look directly into each other's eye

examiner brings in the stimulus—his forefinger—from the periphery

Fig. 4.2 Testing visual fields by confrontation.

obliquely; if the stimulus is moved along a near vertical axis it is difficult to be sure which half of the visual field is being stimulated and large field defects may be missed.

As described, this technique may seem crude and insensitive. In fact it is very reliable; using a pin head as the stimulus very small field defects can be detected. You can prove this for yourself by trying out the method on a colleague and mapping out the scotoma in his visual field produced by the optic nerve head—the normal blind spot.

If the patient is confused or otherwise unable to co-operate, a simple test for a hemianopia can be made by rapidly moving your hand towards the patient's face from one side. This threatening stimulus will usually produce a reflex blink unless the side you have tested is hemianopic.

Ophthalmoscopy

The technique of using the ophthalmoscope takes a good deal of practice to acquire. The best advice is to buy your own instrument and carry it with you so that you can examine the retina and optic disc of every patient that you see without having to rely on the battered equipment in the wards. The optical principle on which the instrument depends is shown in Figure 4.3. From this diagram

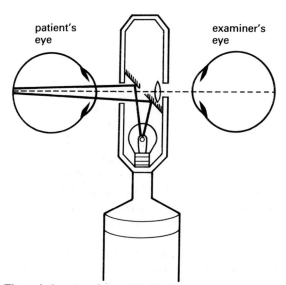

patient's eye

examiner's eye

Fig. 4.3 The optical system of the ophthalmoscope.

you will appreciate that in order to see the patient's retina, three small apertures—your own pupil, the pinhole of the instrument and the patient's pupil—must all fall along the same axis.

Examination

Ask the patient to fix his gaze on a distant object and avoid blocking his view of this point from his other eye while you carry out the examination. This tactic maximizes the chances of his keeping his eye still and thus increases your chances of visualizing the optic fundus. First observe the optic disc: the normal appearance and the changes of papilloedema and optic atrophy are shown diagrammatically in Figure 4.4. Then look at the blood vessels branching from the central retinal artery and vein which enter the eye through the optic nerve. Irregularities in the calibre of the arteries are a sign of arteriosclerosis and, if present, suggest that similar pathology may be affecting other blood vessels in the central nervous system. Sometimes emboli may be seen occluding a retinal artery—another clue about underlying pathology. Ophthalmoscopic features of hypertension or diabetes may be visible. Check too for disease of the retina itself.

THE OCULOMOTOR (III), TROCHLEAR (IV) AND ABDUCENS (VI) NERVES

These are the nerves which innervate the external ocular muscles and are responsible for eye movement. Parasympathetic nerve fibres innervating the sphincter pupillae and the ciliary muscles also travel with the oculomotor nerve.

It is important to know how the six external ocular muscles act to produce movement of the globe of the eye. The actions of the four rectus muscles are easy to understand: the medial rectus moves the eye medially and the lateral rectus moves it laterally; the superior rectus moves the eye to produce upward gaze and the inferior rectus depresses the eye to produce downward gaze. The orbits and the cone formed by the four rectus muscles are obliquely orientated in the skull (Fig. 4.5) so that the superior and inferior recti exert their most powerful action when the eye is looking laterally. By contrast, the other two external ocular muscles, the superior and inferior obliques, work at greatest advantage when the eye is deviated medially. The pull of the oblique muscles is at right angles to the rectus muscles and this

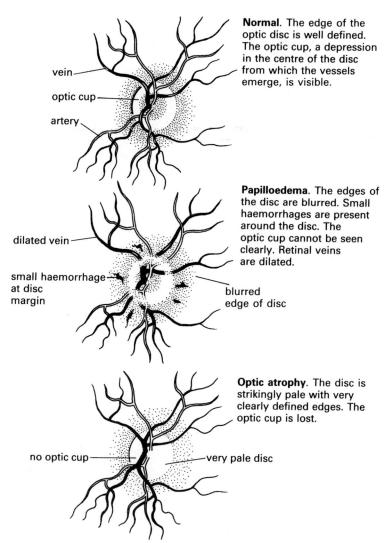

Normal. The edge of the optic disc is well defined. The optic cup, a depression in the centre of the disc from which the vessels emerge, is visible.

vein

optic cup

artery

Papilloedema. The edges of the disc are blurred. Small haemorrhages are present around the disc. The optic cup cannot be seen clearly. Retinal veins are dilated.

dilated vein

small haemorrhage at disc margin

blurred edge of disc

Optic atrophy. The disc is strikingly pale with very clearly defined edges. The optic cup is lost.

no optic cup

very pale disc

Fig. 4.4   Appearances of the optic disc.

means that, when the eye is directed medially, the superior oblique depresses the eye and the inferior oblique elevates it. Figures 4.5 and 4.6 should help to make this clear.

The lateral rectus muscle is innervated by the abducens nerve; the name is logical enough since this is the nerve which abducts the eye. The other rectus muscles and also the inferior oblique

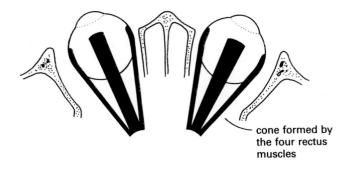

cone formed by
the four rectus
muscles

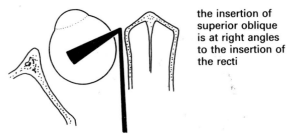

the insertion of
superior oblique
is at right angles
to the insertion of
the recti

Fig. 4.5 Transverse section through the orbits to show the oblique axis of the cone of rectus muscles and the direction of insertion of superior oblique.

are innervated by the oculomotor nerve. The superior oblique is innervated by the trochlear nerve.

Binocular vision depends on the fact that the images formed by the two eyes fall on corresponding parts of the two retinae. It is therefore essential that eye movements are conjugate. If you think for a moment of what happens when you play a game of tennis you will realize the complexities of the neural mechanisms necessary for the maintenance of conjugate gaze. Your opponent lobs the ball; your central nervous system must signal to both sets of external ocular muscles in order to track its trajectory as it rises and falls. As the ball approaches you, the optic axes of the two eyes need to converge, and additional mechanisms are necessary to compensate for the movements of your head and body as you run across the court to position yourself for the smash. The slightest error in the control systems will result in diplopia and your opponent winning the point.

The cortical centre for *voluntary* eye movement is in the frontal lobes anterior to the primary motor cortex. *Tracking* eye move-

When the eye is deviated laterally
superior oblique can only rotate
the eye

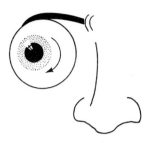

view from
above

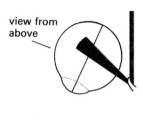

When the eye is deviated medially
superior oblique depresses the eye

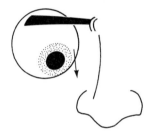

view from
above

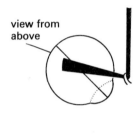

Fig. 4.6   The action of superior oblique.

ments depend on rapid analysis of visual information about the
distance and velocity of the object being followed and are carried
out by areas of visual association cortex close to the primary visual
cortex of the occipital lobes. Both these areas project to the superior colliculi of the mid-brain from which signals are sent to the
nuclei of the three cranial nerves that innervate the external ocular
muscles.

The ability to maintain ocular fixation on a selected target
despite movements of the head, is dependent upon vestibulo-
ocular reflexes. Head movement is detected by the semicircular
canals of the labyrinth. Projections from these organs reach the
oculomotor nuclei via the vestibular nuclei in the brain stem and
cause movement of the eyes to compensate for movement of the
head.

Lateral   gaze   movements   require   collaboration   of   one
oculomotor nerve and the contralateral abducens nerve. For a
conjugate gaze movement to the left, the medial rectus muscle of

the left eye (innervated by the left oculomotor nerve) and the left lateral rectus muscle of the right eye (innervated by the right abducens nerve) must both work in harmony. The nuclei of the oculomotor and abducens nerves communicate by a small but important fibre tract—the median longitudinal bundle (Fig. 4.7). Lesions in this pathway cause a characteristic abnormality in eye movement, an *internuclear ophthalmoplegia*, in which there is incomplete adduction of the eye moving medially and jerking nystagmus of the abducting eye.

When testing eye movements be aware that abnormalities of gaze may be caused not only by lesions in the oculomotor nerves themselves but also by disease of the external ocular muscles, by lesions in the brain stem that affect the oculomotor nuclei and the pathways between them, and by lesions affecting the connections of these nuclei with the vestibular nuclei, mid-brain control centres and cortical visuomotor centres.

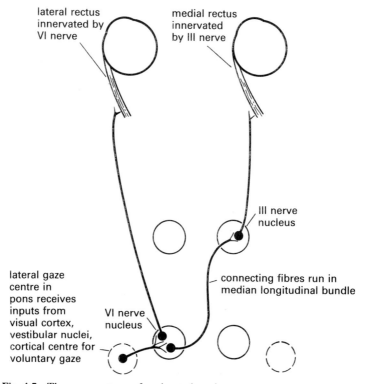

Fig. 4.7   The neuroanatomy of conjugate lateral gaze.

Examination

To test eye movements ask the patient to follow your finger as you move it up and down and from side to side in front of him. Hold his head steady with your other hand. Remember that elderly and middle-aged patients have a near point of at least 30 cm and keep your finger far enough away for him to be able to fixate on it without difficulty (Fig. 4.8). Finally, move your finger towards the patient in order to test his ability to converge his eyes. You should ask the patient to report if he sees double at any stage of the examination.

If you detect any failure of conjugate gaze or the patient reports diplopia you must determine which of the external ocular muscles is failing to work normally. If the defect is gross, simple inspection of the patient's eye movements will provide the answer. More subtle defects require repetition of the examination to determine at which position the two images are maximally separated. Maximum separation of the images occurs when he tries to look in the direction that the defective muscle would normally move the eye and the more peripheral of the two images is derived from the eye into which the defective muscle is inserted. An example may make this clearer; suppose your patient has a palsy of his right abducens nerve and is therefore unable to deviate his right eye laterally. His diplopia will be maximal when he tries to look laterally to the right. When you cover his right eye the more peripheral image will disappear. Figure 4.9 shows why the false image is the more peripheral one. This test sometimes gives unsatisfactory results in

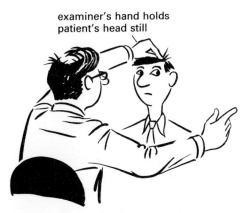

examiner's hand holds
patient's head still

Fig. 4.8 Examination of external ocular movements.

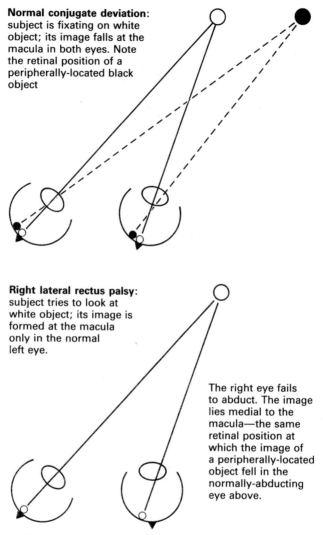

Normal conjugate deviation: subject is fixating on white object; its image falls at the macula in both eyes. Note the retinal position of a peripherally-located black object

Right lateral rectus palsy: subject tries to look at white object; its image is formed at the macula only in the normal left eye.

The right eye fails to abduct. The image lies medial to the macula—the same retinal position at which the image of a peripherally-located object fell in the normally-abducting eye above.

Fig. 4.9 Why the false image is located peripherally in diplopia.

a patient with diplopia of long standing because he has learnt partially to suppress the image from one eye.

The pattern of defective eye movement and other features associated with the ocular palsy should allow you to decide whether the problem lies with the external ocular muscles, the cranial nerves supplying them or the eye movement control centres in the brain stem.

Nystagmus

Nystagmus—rhythmical involuntary movement of the eyes—is a fairly common physical sign but one which causes much unnecessary difficulty in its interpretation. Many people show a few beats on extreme lateral gaze, but nystagmus of clinical significance is almost always sustained and can be elicited within the range of binocular vision. When testing, hold your finger, on which the patient is instructed to fixate, at least 70 cm away so that there is no need for him to converge. Remember to test for nystagmus in both upward and downward directions of gaze as well as horizontally. In practice, of course, this part of the examination is combined with the examination of eye movements.

The direction of the nystagmus may not correspond with the direction of gaze. Vertical nystagmus can occur on lateral gaze and horizontal nystagmus may be present when the patient looks up. Coarse nystagmus is easier to observe than fine nystagmus but both carry the same clinical significance.

Nomenclature

Nystagmus is said to be pendular if the oscillations are of equal speed in both directions, like the swing of a pendulum, rotational if the eye twists about its optical axis and jerking if the oscillations are faster in one direction than the other. Conventionally, jerking nystagmus is further described by the direction of the fast phase of movement. If the eyes drift slowly to the patient's left side and then jerk back to the right, he is said to have jerking nystagmus to the right. (Note that this does *not* mean that the nystagmus is present when the patient looks to his right.) Most people find this convention so difficult to remember that it is far better to describe the nystagmus fully, for example: jerking nystagmus, fast phase to the right, present in all directions of gaze but most marked on lateral gaze to the right.

Types of nystagmus and their significance

Congenital nystagmus

Close inspection reveals a pendular horizontal nystagmus while the patient looks straight ahead, that changes to a jerking horizontal nystagmus on lateral gaze. The nystagmus remains horizontal on up and down gaze. The patient is usually aware that he has the condition and may be quite bored with the disproportionate amount of medical interest displayed. It is usually associated with rather poor visual acuity but is otherwise quite benign.

Vestibular nystagmus

Horizontal jerking nystagmus, often with an additional rotatory component, accompanied by vertigo, nausea, vomiting, tinnitus and deafness is produced by acute labyrinthine failure. There are a number of possible causes: viral infection, thrombotic or embolic occlusion of the labyrinthine artery, trauma and Menière's disease. The fast phase of the nystagmus is away from the affected labyrinth and the nystagmus is increased by gaze in the direction of the fast component.

Benign positional nystagmus

This is a variety of vestibular nystagmus probably caused by degeneration of the otolith organ. The patient experiences vertigo when he holds his head in a particular position, often after he lies down. You can provoke the symptoms by lying the patient flat with his head over the end of the couch slightly below the horizontal and rotated to one side. Nystagmus occurs after a latent period of 15–30 seconds and persists for about half a minute. The patient usually finds this manoeuvre very unpleasant, but, if you can persuade him to let you repeat the test, you will find that the response does not occur a second time.

Central nystagmus

Vertical nystagmus or a combination of vertical and horizontal nystagmus indicates brain stem dysfunction. Localization of the lesion beyond this is often impossible but there is a characteristic syndrome, known as ataxic nystagmus, which consists of horizontal jerking nystagmus in the abducting eye and incomplete adduction of the other eye on lateral gaze and vertical nystagmus on upgaze (Fig. 4.10). Ataxic nystagmus is pathognomic of a lesion in the median longitudinal bundle. Lesions of the cerebellum or its connections with the brain stem produce a horizontal jerking nystagmus most clearly seen on lateral gaze to the side of the lesion.

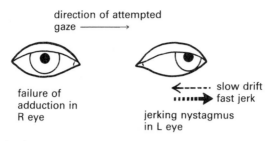

direction of attempted
gaze ──────→

failure of
adduction in
R eye

jerking nystagmus
in L eye

slow drift
fast jerk

Fig. 4.10   Ataxic nystagmus.

Drug-induced nystagmus

Several drugs, including phenytoin, carbamazepine, barbiturates
and alcohol, produce nystagmus of the central type when present
in toxic concentrations—a fact you can verify at any party. A few
drugs, such as gentamicin and streptomycin, are ototoxic and may
cause nystagmus of vestibular origin.

Pupillary reflexes

Light reflex

In response to a light shone in the eye the sphincter pupillae
muscle of the iris constricts. The pathway of the pupillary light
reflex, as this response is called, is shown in Figure 4.11. The afferent limb of the reflex is served by the optic nerve and the efferent limb by parasympathetic nerve fibres from the
Edinger-Westphal nucleus in the mid-brain which travel in the
oculomotor nerve. Normally, both pupils constrict in response to
a light shone in one eye; the ipsilateral response is known as the
direct light reflex and the contralateral response is known as the
consensual light reflex.

By using your knowledge of the anatomy of the reflex you can
work out whether a deficient pupillary reflex is due to a lesion in
the afferent or efferent pathway. For example, if both pupils react
when you shine the light into the left eye but neither respond
when you shine the light into the right eye you can deduce the
presence of a lesion in the afferent pathway on the right; clearly,
because both pupils react when the left eye is stimulated both efferent pathways are working. The lack of response when the right
eye is stimulated can only be caused by a defect in the right optic
nerve. Conversely, if you stimulate the right eye and fail to get a

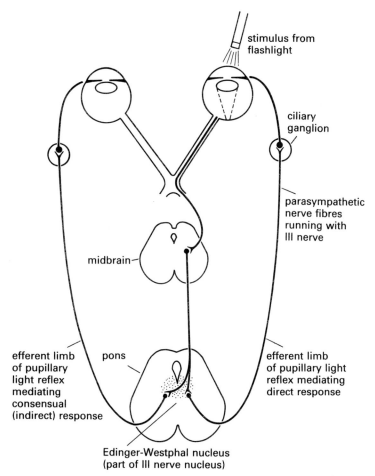

stimulus from
flashlight

ciliary
ganglion

parasympathetic
nerve fibres
running with
III nerve

midbrain

efferent limb
of pupillary
light reflex
mediating
consensual
(indirect) response

pons

efferent limb
of pupillary light
reflex mediating
direct response

Edinger-Westphal nucleus
(part of III nerve nucleus)

Fig. 4.11   The pathway of the pupillary light reflex.

direct response while the consensual response in the left eye is preserved, the lesion must be in the efferent pathway to the right pupil.

Accommodation reflex

When the eyes converge to focus on a nearby object the pupils constrict. The pathway involves centres in the mid-brain and loss of this reflex can occur with expanding lesions of or near the pineal gland which compress the mid-brain lying immediately ventral to

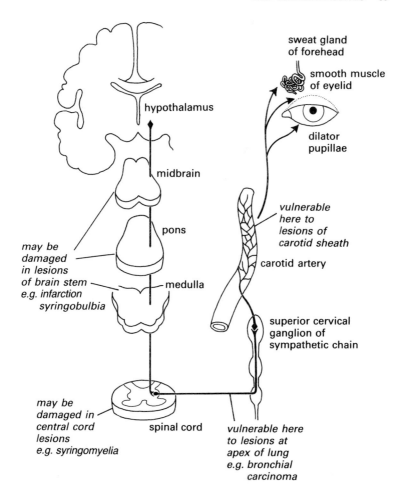

Fig. 4.12 The sympathetic innervation of the eye.

it. Test by getting the patient to focus on your finger held about 15 cm in front of his eyes.

The dilator muscles of the pupil and the tarsal muscles of the upper eye-lid (part of levator palpebrae superioris) are innervated by sympathetic fibres. These fibres pursue a tortuous route to reach the eye and are vulnerable at a number of points (Fig. 4.12). If damaged, a characteristic group of signs—Horner's syndrome—results; there is a partial ptosis, a small pupil and loss of sweating over the ipsilateral part of the face.

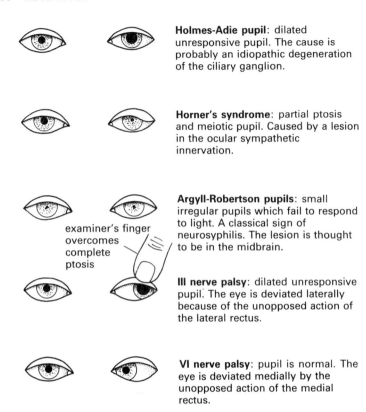

Holmes-Adie pupil: dilated unresponsive pupil. The cause is probably an idiopathic degeneration of the ciliary ganglion.

Horner's syndrome: partial ptosis and meiotic pupil. Caused by a lesion in the ocular sympathetic innervation.

Argyll-Robertson pupils: small irregular pupils which fail to respond to light. A classical sign of neurosyphilis. The lesion is thought to be in the midbrain.

examiner's finger overcomes complete ptosis

III nerve palsy: dilated unresponsive pupil. The eye is deviated laterally because of the unopposed action of the lateral rectus.

VI nerve palsy: pupil is normal. The eye is deviated medially by the unopposed action of the medial rectus.

Fig. 4.13 Common pupillary and ocular abnormalities.

Some of the commoner pupillary and ocular abnormalities found in disease of the nervous system are illustrated in Figure 4.13.

THE TRIGEMINAL (V) NERVE

This nerve has both motor and sensory parts; from the clinical point of view at least, the motor part is far the less important. Let us deal with it first.

Motor

At the rostral end of the main sensory nucleus of the trigeminal nerve is a small motor nucleus. Motor fibres run from this nucleus in the mandibular branch of the nerve to innervate the muscles which open and close the jaw: temporalis, masseter and the pterygoids. The power of these muscles should be tested by asking the patient to clench his teeth and then palpating the masseters and temporalis muscles to assess their tone and bulk. Both these muscles are very strong and weakness must be very profound before it becomes clinically apparent. In contrast, the pterygoids are small muscles and opening the jaw is a relatively weak ·movement. Folklore of the southern states of America has it that an alligator is quite harmless if you grab hold of its snout—the explanation is presumably that its pterygoids are too weak to open its fearsome jaws against the pressure of the hand holding it shut. The human jaw works at less of a mechanical disadvantage and a patient should normally have enough strength to overcome the resistance of a hand pressing upwards against his chin. If the pterygoids are unilaterally weak his jaw will deviate towards the weaker side when he tries to open his mouth. When motor function of the trigeminal nerve is compromised, weakness of opening the mouth may be apparent when it is impossible to detect weakness of jaw closure.

Sensory

The three divisions of the trigeminal nerve supply the face, the inside of the mouth and nasopharynx and the anterior part of the scalp with sensation. Their cutaneous distribution is shown in Figure 4.14. After entering the brain stem, nerve fibres from all three divisions travel caudally for some distance before they synapse, decussate and travel rostrally again alongside the

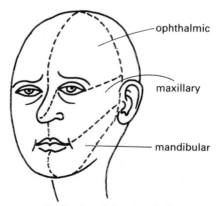

Fig. 4.14   The sensory distribution of the trigeminal nerve.

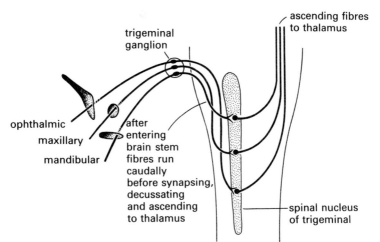

Fig. 4.15   The route taken by sensory fibres of the trigeminal nerve after they enter the brain stem.

spinothalamic tract to reach the thalamus and subsequently the sensory cortex (Fig. 4.15). This anatomical quirk is important because it explains the apparently bizarre pattern of sensory loss that occurs in unilateral medullary lesions. A lesion in the dorsolateral part of the medulla interrupts the descending uncrossed trigeminal fibres and the ascending crossed spinothalamic fibres so that the sensory disturbance affects the ipsilateral half of the face but the contralateral side of the body.

Examination

Testing of trigeminal sensation is performed in the same way as sensation is tested elsewhere on the body using a piece of cotton wool to examine the modality of light touch and a pin to examine pain sensation. Test the corneal reflex too (Fig. 4.16). The cornea of the eye is innervated by the ophthalmic division of the trigeminal nerve. The normal reaction to stimulation of the cornea with a wisp of cotton wool is a blink. Absence of this response indicates a lesion in the trigeminal sensory pathway providing, of course, there is no facial palsy.

The corneal reflex is particularly valuable in testing trigeminal sensation because it is not dependent on the patient reporting how he perceives the stimulus. A patient who claims not to feel touch or pin-prick on his forehead but whose corneal reflex is preserved, is unlikely to have an organic basis for his complaint.

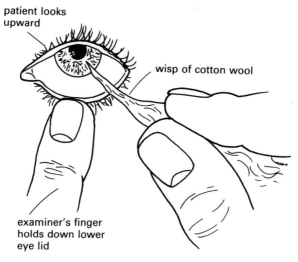

patient looks
upward

wisp of cotton wool

examiner's finger
holds down lower
eye lid

Fig. 4.16 How to test the corneal reflex.

THE FACIAL (VII) NERVE

The facial nerve innervates all the muscles of facial expression. In fact, the only muscles of the face which it does not innervate are the muscles of mastication, which are supplied by the trigeminal nerve, and levator palpebrae superioris, which is supplied by the oculomotor nerve. It also sends motor fibres to a small muscle in the middle ear—stapedius. This muscle damps the oscillations of the ossicles and it contracts reflexly in response to loud noise. Unilateral failure of stapedius to contract causes noises to seem louder on the affected side; this peculiar symptom is known as hyperacusis.

In addition, parasympathetic fibres travelling in the nerve supply the lacrimal gland and the sublingual and submandibular salivary glands. If you are prepared to consider that crying and spitting are also part of the repertoire of facial expressions you may find it easier to remember this component of the facial nerve.

Taste sensation from the anterior two-thirds of the tongue is carried in fibres that travel with the facial nerve for part of its length. Taste fibres exit from the brain stem in the nervus intermedius just next to the motor fibres of the facial nerve. Both nerves run through the internal auditory meatus and pass through the petrous temporal bone but before the motor division of the nerve leaves the skull at the stylomastoid foramen the taste fibres

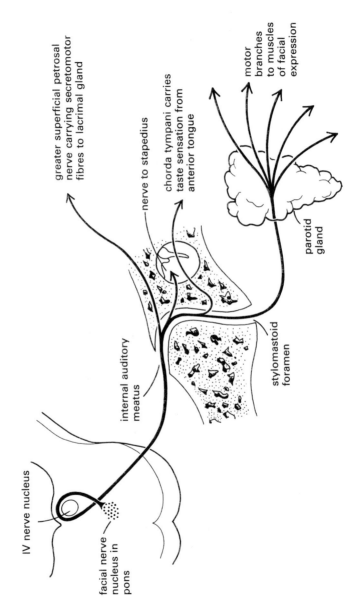

greater superficial petrosal nerve carrying secretomotor fibres to lacrimal gland

nerve to stapedius

chorda tympani carries taste sensation from anterior tongue

motor branches to muscles of facial expression

parotid gland

stylomastoid foramen

internal auditory meatus

IV nerve nucleus

facial nerve nucleus in pons

Fig. 4.17 Diagrammatic representation of the course of the facial nerve.

diverge and pass through the middle ear. This nerve bundle is known as the chorda tympani. If, in a case of a facial nerve palsy, taste is lost, the lesion must be central to the point where the two divisions of the nerve diverge, i.e. within the petrous bone or more proximally. The course of the facial nerve is shown in Figure 4.17.

The upper part of the face is represented bilaterally in the motor cortex. This means that, in lesions of the facial pathway above the facial nerve nucleus, movements of the upper part of the face are preserved. A facial palsy due to an upper motor neurone lesion is therefore restricted to the lower part of the face whereas a lesion of the lower motor neurone causes weakness or paralysis of frontalis and orbicularis oculi as well as the musculature of the lower face. The characteristic appearances of the two types of lesion are shown in Figure 4.18.

Examination

Often a facial palsy can be detected just by looking at the patient's face. The corner of the mouth tends to droop on the affected side and the nasolabial fold is less well-defined. If the lesion is of the lower motor neurone type the patient will be unable to close his eye and the tone of the muscles of the upper and lower eyelids is lost. This leads to inability to blink and a tendency for tears to flow out of the lateral corner of the eye rather than down the lacrimal duct and the patient may look as if he is crying with one eye. In long-standing lesions though, contractures occur and the

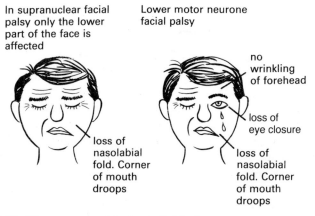

In supranuclear facial palsy only the lower part of the face is affected

Lower motor neurone facial palsy

no wrinkling of forehead

loss of eye closure

loss of nasolabial fold. Corner of mouth droops

loss of nasolabial fold. Corner of mouth droops

Fig. 4.18   The appearance of the face in facial palsy.

asymmetry of the mouth may disappear. Never rely on observation alone to diagnose facial weakness; always test the power of the facial muscles by asking the patient to smile, to puff out his cheeks or to whistle and to screw up his eyes tightly. Try to open his eyes with your fingers while he tries to keep his eyes tightly snut. In a complete facial palsy he will be unable to shut his eye at all but minor degrees of weakness of the upper part of the face can only be detected by testing the power of orbicularis oculi.

When bilateral facial weakness is present the face appears symmetrical although the facial expression is rather lugubrious. Attempts to grin fail to raise the corners of the mouth and produce a 'transverse smile'. A systematic routine of testing the power of facial musculature will prevent bilateral facial weakness being overlooked.

Although the test is not carried out as a routine it is occasionally helpful to examine taste sensation when trying to localize the site of the lesion in a lower motor neurone facial palsy. The patient is asked to protrude his tongue. Using an orange stick with a little cotton wool wrapped around the end, one side of the tongue is moistened with a salty or a sugary solution. Before he puts his tongue back in his mouth, the same solution is applied to the other side of the tongue. The patient is then asked if there is any difference between the two sides. Before repeating the test, allow the patient to rinse his mouth out with water.

THE VESTIBULOCOCHLEAR (VIII) NERVE.

The eighth cranial nerve has two divisions: the vestibular nerve carrying information about the position and movement of the head from the labyrinth and the cochlear nerve which carries auditory information from the cochlear. Peripherally, within the petrous part of the temporal bone, the two divisions travel together. They enter the cranial cavity through the internal auditory meatus, cross the subarachnoid space of the cerebellopontine angle and enter the brain laterally at the junction of the pons and the medulla.

Fibres of the vestibular division synapse in the vestibular nuclei in the lateral part of the medulla and are then distributed to the cerebellum and the nuclei of the cranial nerves controlling the external ocular muscles. Other fibres descend in the vestibulospinal tract. This is a motor pathway to axial musculature that allows the body to compensate for changes in the body's centre of gravity caused by movement of the head. There is also a cortical projection from the vestibular nuclei to the temporal lobe concerned with conscious perception of head position. The extensive connections of the vestibular fibres within the brain stem explain why vertigo and loss of balance are common symptoms in brain stem lesions but the exact details of these pathways are not important.

The central connections of the auditory division of the eighth nerve are complicated. Apart from remembering that there is a bilateral projection to the auditory cortex of the temporal lobe from each cochlear nerve so that central lesions of this pathway very rarely result in deafness, you can forget them. A few fibres from the cochlear nerve run to the facial nerve nucleus and form the afferent limb of the stapedius reflex (see the previous section on the facial nerve). This pathway probably also accounts for the involuntary blink that we make when surprised by a loud noise.

Examination

Test your patient's hearing by occluding one ear with the palm of your hand and whispering a number into the other ear. If you ask the patient to repeat the number that you whispered you can be sure that he really heard it. Always test hearing in both ears. Patients who betray no hint of being hard of hearing while you are taking a history occasionally surprise you by turning out to be profoundly deaf in one ear.

The vestibular division of the nerve cannot really be tested satisfactorily at the bedside though, of course, observation for nystagmus while you are testing eye movements is part of the examination of this nerve. The semicircular canals may be stimulated by irrigating the external auditory meatus with warm or cool water and this produces nystagmus if the nerve is functioning normally. The technique is known as caloric testing and although not difficult to perform its interpretation requires some experience and it cannot be considered as part of the normal clinical examination.

THE GLOSSOPHARYNGEAL (IX) NERVE

This nerve has motor, autonomic and sensory divisions. For all practical purposes the motor and autonomic functions can be ignored. The only muscle supplied by this nerve is stylopharyngeus and its action cannot be tested in isolation because the other muscles that elevate the palate can compensate even when it is completely paralysed. Parasympathetic secretomotor fibres to the parotid gland also run in this nerve but, again, their function cannot easily be tested clinically.

The sensory division supplies the pharynx and the posterior third of the tongue. It also carries taste sensation from the back of the tongue.

Examination

An orange stick may be used to test sensation of the pharynx. The gag reflex, the efferent arm of which is served by the vagus, will be elicited if sensation is normal. The procedure is extremely unpleasant for the patient (if you doubt this try examining your own pharyngeal sensation) and you should reserve this test for those infrequent occasions when it is essential to know that the gag reflex is intact.

THE VAGUS (X) NERVE

This nerve carries the motor supply to the elevators of the palate and the musculature of the pharynx and the larynx. There is a major parasympathetic visceromotor component which innervates the smooth muscle of the respiratory and gastrointestinal tract and the sinoatrial node of the heart. The vagus carries sensation from the larynx, oesophagus and respiratory tract.

Examination

Only a small part of the function of this widely distributed nerve can satisfactorily be tested clinically. Observe that the palate rises symmetrically when the patient phonates; this is most conveniently checked by shining a torch into the patient's open mouth and asking him to say 'aaaaaah'. Get him to cough. The normal cough has an explosive quality which depends on full adduction of the vocal cords to occlude the larynx while intrathoracic pressure is raised, followed by a sudden abduction of the cords to release a blast of air up through the trachea. A lesion of the recurrent laryngeal branch of the vagus precludes complete occlusion of the larynx and the initial explosive part of the cough is lost. Such a cough is often referred to as bovine; listen to a herd of cows going in to be milked on a cold winter's morning to understand why.

THE SPINAL ACCESSORY (XI) NERVE

This nerve is purely motor and is derived from anterior horn cells of the first five cervical segments of the spinal cord. The spinal rootlets join and pass up through the foramen magnum into the skull before exiting through the jugular foramen to supply the sternomastoid muscles and the upper part of trapezius.

Examination

The function of trapezius is tested by asking the patient to shrug his shoulders. Observe that both shoulders rise simultaneously and to the same extent. The sternomastoid rotates the head to the opposite side. Ask the patient to turn his head against resistance provided by your hand on his cheek. Observe and palpate the active muscle (Fig. 4.19).

THE HYPOGLOSSAL (XII) NERVE

This is a purely motor nerve which supplies the intrinsic and extrinsic muscles of the tongue. It leaves the skull through the hypoglossal canal which lies just anterior to the foramen magnum. A unilateral lower motor neurone lesion causes weakness and wasting of the ipsilateral half of the tongue. When the tongue is protruded it deviates toward the weaker side. Fasciculations may be visible; look for these when the tongue is resting on the floor

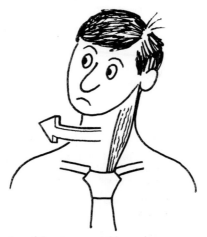

Fig. 4.19 The action of the sternomastoid muscle.

of the mouth. Movements resembling fasciculation can sometimes be seen in normal people when the tongue is protruded and they carry no pathological significance.

Unilateral upper motor neurone lesions cause weakness of the contralateral side of the tongue but there is no accompanying wasting or fasciculation. Bilateral upper motor neurone lesions result in a small spastic tongue which the patient has difficulty in protruding.

Examination

Ask the patient to open his mouth wide and, with the aid of a torch, look for wasting and fasciculations. Ask him to stick his tongue out. Observe whether it is protruded in the midline. If there is any doubt about the presence of a lower motor nerve lesion you can test the strength of lateral movements by getting the patient to put his tongue in his cheek while you press against the outside of his cheek with your fingers.

Table 4.1   Summary of the examination of the cranial nerves

I	Olfactory	Not routinely tested
II	Optic	Test visual acuity, visual fields by the technique of confrontation and observe the retina with an ophthalmoscope
III IV VI	Oculomotor Trochlear Abducens	Test external ocular movements. Note nystagmus or diplopia. Examine the pupillary light and accommodation reflexes
V	Trigeminal	Test the power of jaw opening and closure. Examine sensation over the three divisions of the nerve. Test the corneal reflex
VII	Facial	Observe the face for asymmetry. Ask the patient to smile and to puff out his cheeks. Test the power of eye closure
VIII	Vestibulocochlear	Test hearing in each ear
IX	Glossopharyngeal	Consider whether to test pharyngeal sensation
X	Vagus	Observe palatal movement with phonation. Listen to the patient cough. Consider whether the gag reflex should be tested
XI	Accessory	Test the power of trapezius and sternomastoid muscles
XII	Hypoglossal	Observe the tongue at rest and when protruded

5. The peripheral nerves

The complex structure of a peripheral nerve is illustrated in Figure 5.1. Most nerves contain a mixture of motor, sensory and autonomic nerve fibres, although a few contain only one or two of these fibre types. Individual fibres within a nerve are of various diameters. The largest fibres are myelinated; the smaller fibres run within a Schwann cell but have no myelin sheath. The myelin of the peripheral nervous system is very similar to but not identical with the myelin of the central nervous system. The cell types producing the myelin are different in the two parts of the nervous system. Central nervous system myelin is produced by the oligodendrocyte while the myelin of the peripheral nervous system is produced by the Schwann cell.

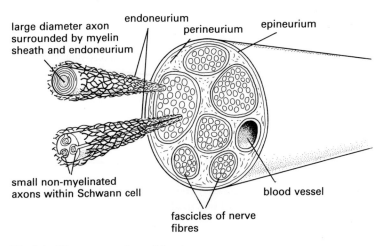

Fig. 5.1 The structure of a peripheral nerve.

PHYSIOLOGY

Conduction of nervous impulses by a propagated action potential is an energy-consuming process and the nerve requires an abundant blood supply. This is provided by small penetrating blood vessels known as the vasa nervorum. In many parts of the body peripheral nerves run alongside arteries and veins forming a neurovascular bundle. Disease of these blood vessels may lead to secondary damage to the accompanying peripheral nerve.

Most of the organelles and enzyme systems responsible for energy production and maintainence of the integrity of the nerve cell are confined to the cell body of the neurone. Providing the long axonal process with the substances it needs to maintain integrity and function poses a formidable transport problem. Some understanding of the size of this problem can be gained by considering a scale model of the nerve cell. Imagine a lower motor neurone in the L5 segment of the spinal cord innervating one of the small muscles in the foot. The length of its axon is of the order of 1 metre and the cell body nourishing this axon is about 50 microns in diameter. If we now want to sketch a diagram of this cell it will be convenient to draw the cell body with a diameter of a couple of centimetres. This represents a linear magnification of about 1000 times. To complete our sketch at the same scale we need to draw an axon of 1 kilometre in length. This simple calculation gives an immediate insight into the symptoms and signs of peripheral neuropathy. Any disease or toxin or metabolic derangement which affects the functions of the nerve cell body is likely to become apparent first at the very distal end of the axon and to affect those nerve cells with the longest axons most severely. Peripheral neuropathies therefore tend to affect the lower limbs before the upper limbs and to affect the distal parts of the limb more severely than the proximal parts.

EFFECTS OF TRAUMA

When a nerve trunk is severed, the axons distal to the disruption degenerate completely. The endoneurial sheaths and the Schwann cells remain. The proximal part of the axons and the nerve cell bodies undergo a number of changes, including the withdrawal of synaptic contacts from other neurones. Regeneration of axons takes place from the proximal stump of the severed nerve by outgrowth of axon sprouts. The functional success of the process of regeneration depends mainly on whether an axon sprout makes contact with its own endoneurial sheath distally. If the correct contact is made the axon sprout can grow again along its previous pathway and the chances of useful reinnervation of the end organ are good. Severe trauma to a nerve trunk damages the distal end of the nerve and disrupts the endoneurial sheaths. Even if axons sprout successfully it is probable that they will grow down the wrong endoneurial sheaths and so make the wrong final connections with the end organs. There will be only limited recovery of function and the aberrant reinnervation may be more of a handicap than a help. Crushing injuries which damage axons but leave the connective tissue skeleton of the nerve intact therefore carry a better prognosis for functional recovery than injuries that cause complete disruption of the nerve trunk. Even so, recovery is delayed many months because the regenerating axons grow at a rate of only a few millimetres each day.

Less severe compression of a peripheral nerve results in mechanical disruption of the myelin sheath and ischaemic damage over a localized segment. Nerve conduction across the affected segment is lost but if the axons remains intact, recovery of function takes place rapidly and is often complete within a few weeks.

DAMAGE TO THE MYELIN SHEATH

The integrity of the myelin sheath is vital for the conduction of impulses by the large nerve fibres. Disruption of this sheath causes peripheral nerve dysfunction just as surely as does damage to the axons themselves. The Schwann cell is vulnerable to certain toxins, e.g. the exotoxin of the organism which causes diphtheria (*Corynebacterium diphtheriae*), acrylamide and some drugs, and also to immunological attack. The commonest form of immunologically mediated demyelination in peripheral nerves is the Guillain-Barré syndrome. This is a subacute condition that initially affects the myelin sheath of motor nerve roots and subsequently extends distally into the peripheral nerve itself. It sometimes follows a trivial respiratory or gastrointestinal infection. The loss of motor function may be so severe and widespread that respiration is affected and ventilatory support required.

EXAMINATION

The function of peripheral nerves is, of course, being tested during the examination of the motor and sensory systems.

Sometimes superficial peripheral nerves may be palpable. Certain types of familial peripheral neuropathy which affect the myelin sheath lead to a recurrent and disorganised sequence of demyelination and remyelination that causes a thickening of the whole nerve trunk. In the inherited condition of neurofibromatosis, multiple peripheral nerve tumours arise. These can often be seen and felt as small, firm, subcutaneous lumps along the course of a peripheral nerve. The most important disease, worldwide, that causes thickening of peripheral nerves is leprosy.

Electrophysiological studies of peripheral nerve function are fairly easy to perform and provide helpful information in the investigation of peripheral neuropathy. These techniques are described in Chapter 15.

6. The autonomic nervous system

Until quite recently, neurologists considered the autonomic nervous system as a rather primitive apparatus that looked after physiological functions below the level of consciousness, like control of motility in the gastrointestinal tract, control of heart rate and maintenance of blood pressure. While it is certainly true that many of the tasks performed by this part of the nervous system are outside conscious control we are beginning to be aware that, far from being primitive, the organization of the autonomic nervous system is exceedingly complicated. Autonomic dysfunction may be a feature of diseases of both peripheral nerves and the central nervous system and may occur as a side-effect of several commonly used drugs. The classical view of the autonomic nervous system divides it into two anatomically and functionally separate parts, the sympathetic and parasympathetic.

THE SYMPATHETIC NERVOUS SYSTEM

Sympathetic fibres of the autonomic nervous system emerge from the thoracic and upper lumbar segments of the spinal cord. The nerve cell bodies of the second order neurones are found in two chains of ganglia which run parallel to and either side of the spinal column. The neurotransmitter of the postganglionic fibres is noradrenalin whose action, broadly speaking, is to cause smooth muscle to contract (α-receptors) and the heart to beat more quickly and more forcefully (β-receptors). There are also non-cardiac β-receptors, designated β_2-receptors, that mediate the relaxation of smooth muscle, especially that of the bronchi.

THE PARASYMPATHETIC NERVOUS SYSTEM

Parasympathetic autonomic fibres emerge from the brain stem and from three sacral segments (S2, 3 and 4) of the spinal cord. The ganglia are located peripherally near the target organs. The postsynaptic transmitter is acetyl choline and its principal actions are to cause smooth muscle to relax, the heart to slow its rate and exocrine glands to secrete.

Figures 6.1 and 6.2 summarize the main functions of the sympathetic and parasympathetic nervous systems.

This dichotomy, although satisfactory for most clinical purposes, is an oversimplification. An increasing number of neurotransmitters and neuromodulators is being identified within the autonomic nervous system and the complex interactions between cholinergic, noradrenergic, peptidergic and probably other transmitter systems (notably serotonin, substance P, VIP and enkephalin) are being investigated. Better understanding of autonomic dysfunc-

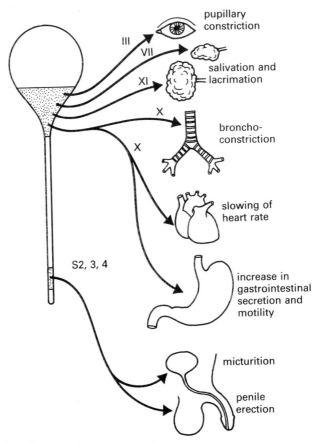

Fig. 6.1 The sympathetic nervous system.

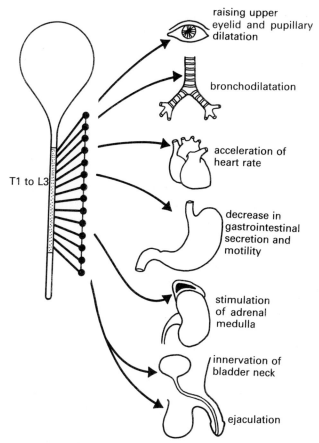

raising upper
eyelid and pupillary
dilatation

bronchodilatation

acceleration of
heart rate

decrease in
gastrointestinal
secretion and
motility

T1 to L3

stimulation
of adrenal
medulla

innervation of
bladder neck

ejaculation

Fig. 6.2   The parasympathetic nervous system.

tion and better methods of treatment of diseases of the autonomic nervous system should result.

The central pathways that control the function of the autonomic nervous system are poorly delineated. The anterior hypothalamus and the brain stem reticular formation are known to be involved and there are also centres within the spinal cord that influence autonomic function.

CLINICAL FEATURES OF AUTONOMIC DYSFUNCTION

Postural hypotension causes feelings of light-headedness or even syncope. The pattern of sweating tends to be abnormal with excessive sweat secretion over the face, upper trunk and arms and decreased secretion over the lower part of the body. Male patients with autonomic dysfunction are usually impotent. There is often hesitancy of micturition and in advanced disease there may be urinary retention. Disturbance of gastrointestinal motility, typically with diarrhoea nocturnally, is also a feature of severe autonomic dysfunction.

Examination

Clinical examination of the autonomic nervous system is rather restricted. Features suggestive of autonomic dysfunction are a sluggish pupillary light reflex and a raised resting heart rate at about 100 to 110 beats per minute. Check too for postural hypotension; a fall of more than about 15 mmHg in systolic blood pressure on moving from a lying to a standing position is abnormal. Painless urinary retention may occur and the abdomen should be palpated for evidence of a distended bladder.

A number of fairly simple tests of autonomic function, which depend on quantitative measures of cardiovascular reflexes, pupillary constriction, bladder function and sweating, can be performed, but these require a certain amount of apparatus and are outside the scope of the clinical neurological examination.

A crude test of sweat function can be made by dusting a thin covering of quinarizine powder or a mixture of starch and iodine powder on the patient's skin and placing him in a warm room, wrapping him with blankets and hot-water bottles and observing the colour change in the powder. When these powders become wet they change colour—to red in the case of quinarizine or to blue-black in the case of starch and iodine.

7. The lobes of the cerebral cortex and higher mental functions

Phrenology, the belief that an individual's mental attributes could be detected by the palpation of bumps on his skull, is now derided as a scientific theory, but it was an important milestone in the history of ideas about localization of function within the cerebral cortex. We no longer believe even in a cortical equivalent of the phrenologist's bump but there is little doubt that particular cerebral functions are localized within particular areas of cortex. Evidence from animal experiments, from direct electrical stimulation of the cortex in unanaesthetized patients and from numerous examples of patients who have sustained injury to localized areas of brain allow us to deduce that certain mental functions depend on the integrity of certain areas of cortex. Localization of function within the various lobes of the cerebral cortex is summarized diagrammatically in Figure 7.1.

The functions of the motor cortex and the sensory cortex, located in the frontal and parietal lobes respectively, were discussed in earlier sections. Speech involves several anatomically distinct regions of the brain and is considered separately in the next chapter. Epilepsy is a frequent result of cortical lesions but this too will be considered separately. In this chapter we are mainly concerned with intellect, mood, memory and will.

THE FRONTAL CORTEX

The famous story of Phineas Gage exemplifies the results of damage to the frontal parts of the cerebral hemispheres. Gage was a foreman employed in the construction of the American railroads. On September 13th 1848 his gang were held up by a formation of rock lying across the planned route of the line. It proved necessary to blast the obstruction and Gage himself took over the business of tamping the charge of gunpowder into a hole drilled

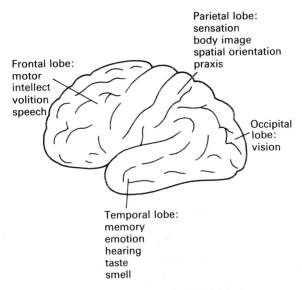

Fig 7.1 Localization of function within the cerebral hemispheres.

into the rock. The tamping iron must have struck a spark from the rock because the charge exploded prematurely. The hole in the rock acted as the barrel of a gun and the tamping iron flew out like a bullet. It entered Gage's head through the roof of his left orbit and came out through the vault of his skull to land many yards away. Amazingly enough, considering the quality of neurosurgical care then available, Gage survived the accident. But his personality was quite changed; he had become mercurial, irresponsible and bad tempered and was quite incapable of foreseeing the consequences of his actions. Unable to continue in his job, he existed by exhibiting himself and the tamping iron at fairgrounds around the country.

This remarkable case-history encapsulates many of the clinical features of frontal lobe injury. A list of these features would include severe intellectual deterioration, disinhibition, an irrepressible tendency to make childish jokes (a phenomenon termed *witzelsucht*), an inability to pursue a purposeful line of action and indifference to personal hygiene and everyday social restraints.

THE TEMPORAL LOBES

In addition to containing the cortical representations of auditory, olfactory and gustatory information, these lobes include the hippo-campal gyri, which are vitally important for memory, and parts of the limbic system, which is concerned with affect and emotion. Our complex behavioural responses to sensory stimuli of all modalities are dependent on the intact functioning of this part of the brain.

Lesions here may produce many different symptoms but the most prominent are loss of memory, alteration in mood and per-sonality, disturbance of emotional responses to pain and pleasure and changes in libido, usually towards hyposexuality but oc-casionally in the other direction.

THE PARIETAL LOBES

The parietal lobes contain the cortical representation of somatic sensation. The role of the primary sensory cortex in the process-ing of sensory information was discussed in the section on sen-sation (see Ch. 3). Adjacent areas of the parietal cortex are involved in the interpretation of that somatosensory input. Lesions here cause loss of the ability to recognize objects by touch even though the patient has no difficulty in actually feeling the object. The spa-tial relationships of the various parts of the object can no longer be integrated to provide a coherent mental picture of the object. Parietal lobe lesions, particularly if they are right-sided, can affect the patient's perception of his own body in a similar way. In the most dramatic cases the patient fails to realize that one side of his body belongs to him and instead forms the idea that the nurses have put someone else's arm or leg in the bed beside him as a macabre practical joke. He may have a distorted idea of the relationship of his body to the space around him, neglecting not only one half of his body but all sensory stimuli, whether tactile, visual or auditory, coming from that side.

Another feature of parietal lobe lesions is loss of the ability to deal with abstract concepts of space. Patients cannot interpret maps and diagrams and cannot produce a copy of a geometrical design. They may also be unable to distinguish left from right. Many normal people, of course, have difficulty with left and right: 'Take the first turn on the right', they say, while simultaneously gesturing with their left arm. Invariably though, it is the verbal label that they get wrong; there is no confusion in their minds about which direction to take. By contrast the patient with a parietal lobe lesion is at a loss where to go. He may get hopelessly lost in surroundings which are quite familiar to him, be quite unable to find the bathroom in his own house for example.

Apraxia is another important feature of parietal lobe lesions. This is the loss of the ability to carry out intentional movements without there being any paralysis of the muscles involved. The patient cannot organize the components of the motor task into the right sequence. In severe cases of apraxia even quite simple sequences of actions may be impossible. Ask a patient to pour and drink a glass of water and he will try to drink from the jug or hold the empty glass to his mouth. Some feeling for what it must be like to be apraxic can be got by remembering what it was like to try to learn a new motor skill yourself. If you have ever tried to ski you will remember your frustration when, while you were falling every few yards, others, with central nervous systems in no way superior to your own, swished past in a series of perfectly executed parallel turns. Your problems were not caused by paralysis or cerebellar dysfunction but by the fact that you couldn't put the necessary muscular contractions together in the right sequence.

The terms ideomotor and ideational are sometimes applied to different forms of apraxia and you may come across them in textbooks. It is usually very difficult to understand quite what these terms mean from the definitions given and, in any case, they are often used inconsistently. Indeed the actual existence of different forms of apraxia is the subject of controversy. I suggest that you ignore these categories. One term that you should be familiar with is *dressing apraxia*; this refers, obviously enough, to confusion about the sequence of actions needed to put clothes on. Patients with this disorder become quite muddled about the order in which garments should be put on, how they should be put on and which parts of the body they should cover. This is probably just one manifestation of apraxia rather than a specific category of the disorder.

Lateralization of function in the parietal lobes is the subject of much argument among psychologists. Right-sided lesions (i.e. lesions in the non-dominant hemisphere) tend to produce sensory inattention to the left, problems with the interpretation of spatial relationships and apraxia which affects mainly the limbs on the left side of the body. Left-sided parietal lobe lesions often produce apraxia which affects both sides of the body.

THE OCCIPITAL LOBES

The occipital lobes are entirely concerned with the processing of visual information. A unilateral lesion in the primary visual cortex will result in a contralateral homonomous visual field defect. The reason for this will be obvious if the anatomy of the visual pathways is understood (see Fig. 4.1).

The primary visual cortex is located along the medial surfaces of the two occipital lobes and at their posterior pole. Adjacent on the lateral surfaces are the visual association cortices where higher level analysis of visual input is undertaken. Localized lesions of this area can result in bizarre distortions of visual perception. Objects may seem too large or too small, or very close or very distant as if viewed down the wrong end of a telescope. The shape of objects may be distorted or they may persist in the visual field after gaze has been shifted away. A re-reading of *Alice in Wonderland* will provide excellent examples of the results of dysfunction of visual association cortex.

If lesions of the visual association cortex extend anteriorly into the temporal lobes, a deficit known as visual agnosia may be present. Although the object is seen its significance is not appreciated. It cannot be named, recognized or used properly. The defect may be confined to a particular class of visual stimuli; one example is failure to recognize other people by their facial appearance—*prosopagnosia*—though they can be recognized by their voice. These abnormalities of visual perception are not common, but too often patients with these symptoms are treated for a psychiatric disorder because the organic nature of the lesion is not realized.

Although the emphasis of this chapter has been on the localization of particular functions to specific areas of cortex you should be aware that even the most mundane of activities is likely to require the simultaneous and integrated action of many parts of the cortex. While you walk down the ward (motor activity) to clerk in a new patient (language) you remember to collect an ophthalmoscope (memory) and open the cupboard to find it (sequence of intentional muscular movements and visual recognition of object) while, all the time, you are thinking how much nicer it would be to be outside playing tennis (emotion). Deficits in any one cortical function may well have secondary effects on other cortical activities. It is important to realize too, that diseases of the nervous system may not respect boundaries between different areas of cortex and that deficits in many aspects of higher mental function may be present simultaneously.

CLINICAL EXAMINATION OF HIGHER MENTAL FUNCTION

Before starting try to obtain some information about the patient's premorbid personality and intellectual function. This will allow you to estimate how well he ought to perform in the tests. Establish too, that the patient is not dysphasic; if he has difficulties with language he will obviously have difficulty with any tests requiring verbal skills.

Orientation

Ask the patient where he is, what sort of building he is in, who the people around him are, what day of the week it is, what month and year it is.

Memory

Give the patient a fictitious name and address to remember. Make sure that he can repeat it back immediately and then continue with other tests. A few minutes later ask him if he can recall the name and address that you gave him earlier.

An alternative, slightly harder, test of memory is the Babcock sentence: 'There is one thing a nation must have to be rich and great and that is a large, secure supply of wood'. The sentence should be repeated alternately by the examiner and the patient until two word-perfect recitations have been obtained. Give up if, after eight repetitions, he is unable to learn it. Test recall a few minutes later.

Avoid the common mistake of testing memory by asking what the patient had for breakfast. Quite apart from the fact that many normal but non-gastronomically orientated people forget what they have eaten soon after a meal, you have no way of knowing whether his answer is correct or whether he is confabulating.

Intellect and concentration

Ask him if he knows the proverb, 'A stitch in time saves nine'. Ask

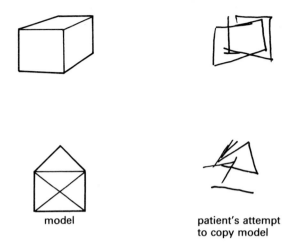

model   patient's attempt
                         to copy model

Fig. 7.2   Examples of drawings by patients with lesions affecting the parietal lobe.

him to explain what it means. Patients with intellectual deterioration tend to paraphrase and produce a very literal interpretation instead of extracting a generalized meaning.

Test his knowledge of current events. Who is the Prime Minister? What is in the news at the moment?

Ask him to subtract 7 from 100, and then to continue subtracting 7 from what is left. Most people can complete this test in less than a minute with only one or two mistakes.

Tests for apraxia

The patient should be asked to draw a clock face and indicate a time on it. He can also be asked to copy simple designs. Figure 7.2 shows some examples drawn by patients with parietal lobe lesions.

Other tests for apraxia include asking the patient to perform motor tasks to order. These can be improvised as necessary: make a fist, point with your left index finger, show me how you would comb your hair, mime someone playing the violin.

8. Disorders of speech

A patient rendered unable to communicate by neurological disease, especially if the disorder has been of sudden onset, is in a most bewildering and frustrating situation. The very least you can do for him is to make an accurate diagnosis, assess the extent of his disability fully and show him that you are aware of and understand his difficulty. This is not a hard thing to do. There are only four reasons why he may not be able to speak: he may be *dysphonic*, *dysarthric*, *dysphasic* or, just possibly, *mute*.

DYSPHONIA

In order to produce any volume of speech it is necessary to move air from the lungs past tense vocal cords to create resonant frequencies in the same way that musical instruments produce sound when air is blown past a reed. The resonance is subsequently modulated into comprehensible speech by changes in shape of the cavities of the pharynx and mouth. Disease of the larynx or defects in the innervation of the vocal cords will prevent the larynx performing this function. The presence of a tracheostomy causes dysphonia because air can no longer reach the vocal cords and set them vibrating. The patient will appear to be mouthing words but no sound will be heard. Minor degrees of dysphonia are apparent only as hoarseness or an inability to speak loudly. Occasionally, dysphonia is hysterical or a manifestation of extreme anxiety—you may have experienced a transient dysphonia yourself if you have ever had to speak in public—but this functional complaint is easy to diagnose because the ability to cough is preserved (see p. 74, concerning the vagal innervation of the larynx).

DYSARTHRIA

Frequent, rapid and precise movements of lips, tongue, jaw and palate are necessary for clearly articulated speech. Dysarthria is the name given to disorders of speech resulting from defective movements of these structures. Words are not enunciated distinctly and consonant sounds are slurred.

There are a number of characteristic types of dysarthria which are usually fairly easy to distinguish.

Cerebellar dysarthria

Speech has an explosive quality, a sort of verbal equivalent of intention tremor, because the patient cannot control the volume accurately. Some syllables and words are spoken too loudly, others too softly. Timing of speech is also affected so that sentences are spoken in a jerky and staccato fashion. This is sometimes known as scanning dysarthria, presumably by analogy with the way in which syllables are overemphasized when a line of verse is scanned aloud to demonstrate the metre.

Spastic dysarthria

Bilateral upper motor neurone lesions affecting the lower cranial nerves cause weakness and spasticity of the muscles of the tongue and pharynx. The patient has particular difficulty in pronouncing the plosives 'b', 'p', 't', and 'd'. Palatal movement may also be restricted, which gives a nasal quality to speech. The overall effect is of the patient speaking from the back of his mouth without moving the tip of the tongue or his lips. The voice in spastic dysarthria sounds a bit like that of the Disney cartoon character Donald Duck.

Dysarthria of Parkinson's disease

The rigidity and bradykinesia of this condition result in very monotonous speech which is devoid of expression or inflection. Speech is quiet and the words tend to run into one another. In severe cases the patient may have difficulty in starting a word, particularly at the beginning of a sentence, and the first syllable is repeated over and over again—a phenomenon known as *pallilalia*.

Dysarthria of myasthenia gravis

The characteristic feature of the muscle weakness in myasthenia gravis is fatiguability. This is manifested in speech by gradual loss of volume and clarity. The sentence starts normally but soon the voice becomes softer, hoarser and acquires a nasal quality. After a short period of rest, or an injection of the short-acting cholinesterase inhibitor edrophonium, the voice returns to normal.

DYSPHASIA

Dysphasia is the name given to conditions in which formulation or comprehension of language is impaired. The cause is always a lesion of the dominant cerebral hemisphere and it is therefore an important localizing sign. Language function is located in the left hemisphere of all right-handed individuals and probably in 50–60% of left-handers too. Of the remaining left-handers, about half have language represented bilaterally and half have it located exclusively in the right hemisphere. There are a number of classifications of dysphasia in current use that you may encounter. Most have been designed primarily for neuropsychological research and are unnecessarily complex for clinical use. The categories described below are quite adequate for most clinical purposes.

Expressive dysphasia

This type of dysphasia is also known as motor dysphasia or Broca's dysphasia because it is caused by lesions in the posterior inferior part of the frontal lobe—Broca's area (Fig. 8.1). The lesion affects the capacity for expression in the form of language. In its most profound form there is no speech at all. In slightly less severe cases simple words like 'yes' or 'no' may be spoken, although not always appropriately. In milder cases there is a reduction in the amount of spontaneous speech and descriptive words, adjectives and adverbs are left out. Only the most essential words for preservation of meaning are used so that the content of speech resembles the wording of a telegram. Automatic speech, like the recitation of nursery rhymes or counting from 1 to 20, is usually remarkably intact and the patient may be able to sing without difficulty. Despite these problems of expression the patient's comprehension of spoken language is intact.

Receptive dysphasia

Synonyms for this form of dysphasia are Wernicke's dysphasia or central dysphasia. The lesion involves Wernicke's area in the superior middle and posterior regions of the temporal lobe immediately inferior to the region of cortex concerned with auditory reception (Fig. 8.1). In contrast to expressive dysphasia the patient's difficulty is in the comprehension of speech. He is unable to understand his own speech or that of others. He can produce words and sentences but, because he has lost the ability to monitor his own speech output, much of what he says is gobbledegook. He may substitute a wrong but related word, e.g. table for chair, or he may produce meaningless jargon. These meaningless inventions are known as *neologisms* and the whole fluent but unintelligible output is sometimes referred to as jargon dysphasia or word salad.

Global dysphasia

Many patients with dysphasia do not fit clearly into either of the above two categories. They have difficulty with both comprehension and expression. Extensive lesions of the dominant hemisphere often leave patients literally speechless and with profound difficulties in understanding language. Such a condition is termed global dysphasia.

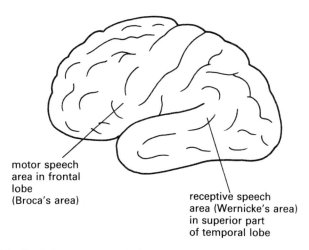

motor speech
area in frontal
lobe
(Broca's area)

receptive speech
area (Wernicke's area)
in superior part
of temporal lobe

Fig. 8.1   Cortical areas concerned with speech.

Nominal dysphasia

This form of dysphasia, known also as anomic or amnesic dysphasia, is a specific difficulty in finding the names of objects. The patient is able to comprehend spoken language without trouble and can express himself in well-constructed sentences. He may be able to disguise his difficulty with naming by circumlocution and, if the deficit is mild, it may go undetected in everyday conversation. Show him an everyday object, a comb for example, and he will demonstrate that he knows exactly what it is but ask him to name it and he will resort to '. . . the thing you use to tidy your hair'. If he is prompted by a series of nouns—'Is it a pen? Is it a banana? Is it a hammer?'—he will reject the wrong names but he will not always recognize the right one.

Nominal dysphasia is quite frequently found in patients who have recovered from a more severe expressive dysphasia. As an isolated phenomenon it is said to indicate a lesion in the dominant posterior temporoparietal region, but it is frequently found in cases where there is more diffuse cerebral damage. Read the novel *Ending Up* by Kingsley Amis, in which the character George suffers from nominal dysphasia, to gain an impression of what it is like to suffer from this disability.

MUTISM

Patients with severe expressive or global dysphasia may be mute in the sense that they utter no words at all. Occasionally patients, usually preadolescent boys from disturbed backgrounds, without any organic brain lesion decide to forego all verbal communication—a condition known as *elective mutism*.

EXAMINATION OF SPEECH

Language problems of any severity will usually become obvious soon after you meet the patient and start to take the history. Dysphonia is immediately apparent and the examination should centre on the larynx and its innervation. In severe cases of pseudobulbar or bulbar palsy, where the laryngeal and pharyngeal musculature is completely paralysed, the patient will be completely aphonic and anarthric and therefore unable to produce any intelligible sound. If examination of the lower cranial nerves is neglected the patient may be wrongly diagnosed as having expressive dysphasia.

Minor degrees of dysarthria can be clarified by asking the patient to repeat the time-honoured tongue-twisters, 'West Register Street' and 'Peter Piper picked a peck of pickled peppers' while you listen carefully to the pronounciation of the 'p' and 't' sounds. If you suspect myasthenia you can ask the patient to count or recite a nursery rhyme in order to bring out the fatiguing of the voice. The type of dysarthria will point out the next step in the examination. If speech is staccato or scanning, suspect a cerebellar lesion and examine for other cerebellar signs. If the patient is unable to pronounce 'b', 'p', 'd' and 't' and sounds as if he is speaking from the back of his mouth, your attention should be directed at the lower cranial nerves to look for signs of a pseudobulbar palsy. Soft, monotonous speech in which the individual words are run together suggests a diagnosis of parkinsonism.

Before analysing dysphasia, try to obtain some information about the patient's native language and background. Your reputation as a diagnostician will not be enhanced if you make a confident diagnosis of fluent receptive dysphasia in a patient who turns out to be an East European unable to speak English.

Start by observing spontaneous speech. Is it fluent? Does it contain neologisms or inappropriate words? Does the patient use descriptive words or is his speech telegraphic?

Check for receptive dysphasia by giving the patient a set of clear instructions that can be obeyed without needing a verbal response. Ask him, for example, to raise his right hand or to shut his eyes. If these simple commands are performed correctly increase the complexity of the task: 'Fold this sheet of paper in half and then place it on the table in front of you'.

Ask the patient to name objects: show him things like a pen, a watch and your stethoscope. Make it more difficult by requiring him to itemize the component parts of the object such as the clip and the nib of the pen.

Try finally to decide whether the dysphasia is expressive or receptive, or whether both aspects of language function are impaired.

9. Examination of the unconscious patient

Loss of consciousness occurs as a non-specific response to a wide range of insults to the central nervous system and has no localizing value as a clinical sign. It is true, of course, that consciousness depends on having a functioning cerebral cortex and that the cortex relies on a constant stream of impulses arriving from the ascending reticular formation in the brain stem to keep it awake, but all that can be deduced from this in an unconscious patient is that either the cortex or the brain stem or both have ceased to function normally.

The first priority when confronted with an unconscious patient is to ensure that he is removed from imminent danger, that he is breathing and his airway is clear and that he has an adequate cardiac output. Resuscitation must precede diagnosis.

The essential clue to the reason for the patient's reduced level of consciousness is often obtained from information about the circumstances in which he was found. Relatives, onlookers, the police or ambulance men frequently provide vital facts about trauma, drug-overdose, alcohol intake and medical history. His general practitioner can probably be reached by telephone; his knowledge of the patient may be helpful.

A list of causes of unconsciousness is given in Table 9.1.

ASSESSMENT OF LEVEL OF CONSCIOUSNESS

The progress of an unconscious patient and his eventual prognosis can be determined by serial assessments of how deeply he is unconscious. If his conscious level is improving it is unlikely that any urgent intervention is necessary and his prognosis for recovery is good. A deepening level of unconsciouness by contrast may call for immediate action. It is clearly essential, if repeated estimations

Table 9.1   Causes of unconsciousness

Metabolic	Hypothermia
	Hypoglycaemia
	Diabetic ketoacidosis
	Other acid-base disturbances
	Hypothyroidism
	Hypoadrenalism
	Hypopituitarism
	Hepatic failure
	Renal failure
Drugs	Alcohol
	Hypnotics
	Tricyclic antidepressants
	Aspirin, etc.
Anoxia	Respiratory failure
	Cardiac arrest
	CO poisoning
Infection	Meningitis
	Encephalitis
	Cerebral abscess
	Systemic infection
Primary intracranial	Intracerebral haemorrhage
	Subarachnoid haemorrhage
	Subdural haematoma
	Extradural haematoma
	Cerebral infarction
	Brain stem infarction or haemorrhage
	Cerebral trauma
	Cerebral neoplasm
Epilepsy	Status epilepticus
Hypertensive encephalopathy	

of conscious level are to have any value, for the method of assessment to be as free of interobserver variation as possible and for the terms in which conscious level is described to be unambiguous. For these reasons terms such as stupor, coma or obtundation are inadequate. Numerical scales have been developed to surmount these difficulties. The Glasgow Coma Scale, which is described below, has been well validated and shown to be easy to use and reliable.

The Glasgow Coma Scale

This scale gives a numerical score to the patient's conscious level from observations of the patient's behaviour. The method of scor-

Table 9.2   The Glasgow Coma Scale

Test	Score
Eye opening	
Eyes open spontaneously	4
Eyes open when the patient is spoken to	3
Eyes open in response to painful stimuli	2
Eyes do not open at all	1
Best verbal response	
Patient shows that he is orientated	5
Patient is confused	4
Patient uses inappropriate words	3
Patient utters incomprehensible sounds	2
No sounds uttered at all	1
Best motor response (usually recorded from the better arm)	
Patient will obey commands	5
Patient makes a co-ordinated response to a painful stimulus	4
The patient's limb flexes to a painful stimulus	3
The patient's limb extends to a painful stimulus	2
No response to a painful stimulus	1
Maximum total	14

ing is shown in Table 9.2. The assessment is easy to perform and the results are simple to record. Many wards have printed forms to allow the charting of serial observations.

The Glasgow Coma Scale is not intended to be a substitute for the neurological examination of an unconscious patient but it is a very valuable adjunct to it.

EXAMINATION OF THE UNCONSCIOUS PATIENT

Start by checking the patient's vital signs: temperature, pulse rate, blood pressure and respiratory rate. Look at the skin for evidence of cyanosis or the presence of a rash. Smell his breath for foetor hepaticus or ketones. Examine the head and neck for signs of trauma. An auriscope must be used to examine the external auditory meatus for signs of middle ear infection and for evidence of leakage of blood or of cerebrospinal fluid. Inspect the nose for CSF leakage.

Examine for neck stiffness and Kernig's sign (Fig. 9.1). If present these signs suggest meningeal irritation caused either by subarachnoid blood or infection and inflammation of the meninges. Herniation of the cerebellar tonsils into the foramen magnum is a less

A

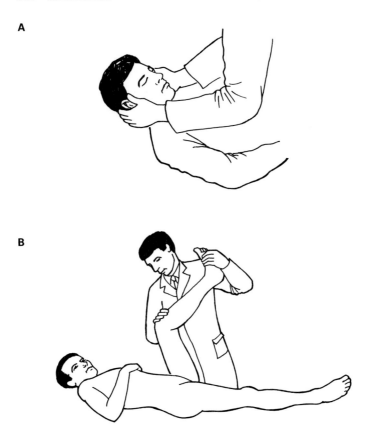

B

Fig. 9.1 How to examine for meningeal irritation. **A** Testing for neck stiffness. The patient should normally be able to reach the sternum with his chin. **B** Kernig's sign. Attempts to extend the knee when the hip is flexed evoke spasm in the hamstrings.

common cause of neck stiffness. A very rare cause of neck stiffness, but one that it is essential not to overlook, is tetanus.

A complete assessment of the cranial nerves is not feasible, but this is not a reason for not examining them as fully as possible. Pay particular attention to the ophthalmoscopic examination of the optic nerve head to look for evidence of raised intracranial pressure. Examine also the size and equality of the pupils and their reaction to light, whether conjugate gaze is preserved and if the eyes are deviated to one or other side, whether reflex eye movements are present in response to turning the patient's head from side to side, whether nystagmus is present, whether the corneal reflex is preserved and whether there are any spontaneous gagging, coughing or swallowing movements.

There is no difficulty in examining muscle tone, but remember that in acute pyramidal tract lesions tone may be reduced rather than increased on the affected side. By lifting a limb and letting it fall it may be possible to identify a hemiplegia. A paralysed limb drops back to the bed like a stone but in the absence of paralysis, except in the most profoundly unconscious patients, the fall is checked.

Tendon reflexes can be elicited in the usual way. The plantar responses are almost invariably extensor no matter what the cause of unconsciousness.

Beyond testing the response to a painful stimulus, which is best delivered by pressing on the patient's finger or toe nail with the tip of your own thumbnail, no useful assessment of sensation is possible.

Investigations

Because of the urgency of making a diagnosis and the inadequacy of the history and examination in most unconscious patients, radiological and laboratory investigations are often essential.

Plasma electrolyte and glucose concentrations

A number of metabolic abnormalities and endocrine deficiencies may present as coma and all unconscious patients should have blood taken for immediate analysis of plasma electrolyte and glucose concentrations. It is, of course, essential that blood is drawn before any intravenous fluid therapy is started. Blood gas analysis is essential if there is any suspicion of acid–base disturbance or of ventilatory failure. Toxicological screening is often needed; one of the commonest causes of unconsciousness in young people is deliberate self-poisoning.

CT scanning

This is invaluable in the management of unconsciousness caused by trauma. Extradural and subdural haematomas can be diagnosed with a high degree of certainty and treated without delay. Many other intracranial causes of unconsciousness can be diagnosed accurately by this means and, even if neurosurgical intervention is not appropriate, management plans can be made rationally.

Lumbar puncture

Examination of the CSF is essential whenever meningitis is suspected. It may also be valuable to confirm a diagnosis of subarachnoid haemorrhage. In certain circumstances, notably raised intracranial pressure due to a space-occupying lesion in the posterior fossa, lumbar puncture may be disastrous for the patient. If there is any doubt about the safety of the procedure a CT scan should be undertaken first.

Electroencephalography

In cases of status epilepticus, particularly if the seizures are not generalized—non-convulsive status—an EEG may be the only way of confirming the diagnosis and the response to treatment. This condition is discussed more fully in Chapter 16.

THE LOCKED-IN SYNDROME

Very rarely, bilateral lesions of the ventral part of the pons result in a syndrome of total quadriplegia with additional paralysis of facial and bulbar musculature. The patient's conscious level may be unimpaired but, because almost all efferent pathways have been destroyed, he is unable to react to external stimuli by speech or movement of limbs or face. The only voluntary movements left to him are those mediated by the external ocular muscles and it is only by eye movement, and sometimes by opening and shutting his eyelids, that he can signal to an observer.

This condition is known as the locked-in syndrome and it can easily be mistaken for unconsciousness if the examination does not include asking the patient to open and shut his eyes and testing external ocular movements.

The underlying pathology is either infarction secondary to basilar artery occlusion or massive demyelination and the prognosis is extremely poor. However, it is obviously very important that a patient afflicted with this awful condition is not treated as though he were unconscious.

BRAIN DEATH

The success of modern techniques of resuscitation and intensive care allows a number of patients with irreversible damage to the brain stem to survive. The word survive is used only in the sense that continued artificial ventilation of these patients allows the heartbeat to continue. When all brain stem function is permanently lost, no possibility of recovery of any cerebral function remains. In such circumstances the patient may be declared brain dead, ventilation discontinued and a death certificate issued.

Strict criteria for a diagnosis of brain death have been formulated.

Preconditions for a diagnosis of brain death

There must be a positive diagnosis of the cause of the patient's irreversible brain damage. Common causes are severe head injury, massive intracerebral haematoma and anoxic brain damage.

The possibility that the patient's condition is due to drugs with a depressive activity on cerebral function, hypothermia, or metabolic or endocrine disturbance must be excluded.

The patient must be apnoeic and there must be no possibility that neuromuscular blocking agents are responsible for the apnoea.

Testing for absence of brain stem reflexes

There is no pupillary reaction to a bright light shone in either eye.

No reaction is obtained to attempts to elicit the corneal reflex.

No eye movements occur in response to the slow injection of 50 ml of ice-cold water into either external auditory meatus.

There is complete absence of gag, swallow or cough reflexes in response to bronchial stimulation.

No facial motor response is obtained to a painful stimulus, such as pressure on the superior margin of the orbit.

Testing for apnoea

No respiratory movements are observed when the patient is disconnected from the ventilator.

To ensure that there is an adequate hypercapnic stimulus to respiration 5% carbon dioxide is added to the inspired air before the test is performed and blood gases are checked. An arterial P_{CO_2} of 6.8 kPa or greater is required. To avoid endangering the patient by anoxia during the test, oxygen is given by an endotracheal cannula at 6 l/min.

Conditions of testing

The tests for brain death should be carried out by two doctors, either individually or together. Both doctors should be experienced and of either senior registrar or consultant grade. The tests should be repeated after an interval. Usually 12 to 24 hours are allowed to pass between the two tests.

10. The general examination: items of special relevance to neurological disease

A number of aspects of the general medical examination take on particular importance and significance in a patient who presents with neurological symptoms. Vital clues to a primary disease of the nervous system may be found in other systems. For example, the presence of adenoma sebaceum in the skin of a patient presenting with epilepsy points to an underlying diagnosis of tuberose sclerosis. Conversely, neurological symptoms may have their explanation in a disease of another system. For example, a patient who presents with loss of consciousness may have aortic stenosis.

A brief summary of some of the physical signs found on general examination that may point to a diagnosis of neurological disease is given below.

Table 10.1 Physical signs which may indicate disease of the nervous system

Physical sign	Possible neurological implication
Facial appearance	
Lack of facial expression	Bradykinesia of Parkinson's disease
	Bilateral facial weakness
Ptosis	Horner's syndrome
	Myasthenia gravis
	Partial III nerve palsy
Exophthalmos	Thyrotoxicosis (neurological presentations include proximal myopathy and tremor)
	Retro-orbital tumour
Hairless appearance	Hypopituitarism
Butterfly rash	Systemic lupus erythematosus
Acromegalic face	Pituitary tumour
Coarse puffy facial features	Hypothyroidism (neurological presentations include carpal tunnel syndrome, other entrapment neuropathies, proximal myopathy and cerebellar degeneration)
	Long-term treatment with phenytoin

Table 10.1 *(cont'd)*

Physical sign	Possible neurological implication
Skin	
Cafe au lait patches	Neurofibromatosis
Cutaneous neurofibromata	Neurofibromatosis
Adenoma sebaceum	Tuberose sclerosis
Finger clubbing	
	Carcinoma of the bronchus (possibility of cerebral or cerebellar secondaries)
	Chronic pulmonary sepsis (may cause cerebral abscess)
	Cyanotic congenital heart disease (which causes secondary polycythaemia and increased risk of thrombosis and embolism)
Goitre or thyroidectomy scar	
	Thyroid disease (associated with myasthenia gravis and dystrophia myotonica)
Abdomen	
Enlarged liver	Alcoholic liver disease (neurological presentations include peripheral neuropathy, myopathy, Wernicke's encephalopathy, dementia, and hepatic encephalopathy)
	Wilson's disease
	Metastatic carcinoma
Enlarged spleen	Polycythaemia (neurological presentations include cerebral thrombosis and embolism)
Cardiovascular system	
Rhythm disturbance	Cerebral emboli
	Autonomic neuropathy
Valvular disease	Infectious endocarditis (neurological presentations include cerebral abscess and embolism)
	Mitral stenosis (cerebral embolism)
	Aortic stenosis (loss of consciousness)
Systemic hypertension	Cerebrovascular disease
Arterial bruits	Cerebrovascular disease

Neurological investigations

11. Examination of cerebrospinal fluid

Examination of the CSF is indicated for three main reasons:

1. In case of suspected meningitis or encephalitis to confirm the clinical diagnosis and identify the responsible organism.
2. To confirm a clinical diagnosis of subarachnoid haemorrhage.
3. To aid the diagnosis of other neurological diseases, especially multiple sclerosis and neurosyphilis.

Specimens of CSF for analysis are usually obtained by lumbar puncture, although under special circumstances they can also be taken from the cisterna magna or directly from the cerebral ventricles. Lumbar puncture is sometimes performed for reasons other than to obtain CSF for diagnostic purposes. The procedure allows the pressure of CSF in the subarachnoid space to be measured or contrast medium to be introduced for radiological purposes.

Lumbar puncture is potentially dangerous in cases of raised intracranial pressure, particularly if the increased pressure is caused by the presence of a space-occupying lesion. Puncturing the dura creates a hole through which CSF can leak. Leakage increases the pressure gradient in the CSF between intracranial and spinal compartments and may precipitate downward herniation of brain through the tentorium or the foramen magnum with lethal consequences. If there is any reason to suspect raised intracranial pressure do not carry out a lumbar puncture until other investigations, which probably need to include a CT scan of the head, have shown that it is safe to do so.

THE TECHNIQUE OF LUMBAR PUNCTURE

Explain to your patient what you are going to do in an honest but reassuring way. Lumbar puncture should not be a painful experience but generations of ham-fisted doctors have ensured that it has a reputation among the lay public for causing excruciating agony.

Position the patient on the edge of the bed comfortably curled up into a fetal position. In this position the interlaminar spaces are as widely separated as possible. The patient's back should be perpendicular so that the spine is not rotated. The correct positioning of the patient is shown in Figure 11.1.

Identify the L3/4 and L4/5 interspaces. A line joining the iliac crests passes through the body of the fourth lumbar vertebra. The L3/4 and L4/5 interspaces are situated immediately above and below this line and provide the largest target for the spinal needle.

Clean and drape the area. Inject a few millilitres of local anaesthetic just underneath the skin at the point where you plan to insert the spinal needle.

Check that you have all the necessary equipment: manometer, three-way tap for connecting the manometer to the needle and three sterile containers for the collection of CSF.

Insert a 20-gauge spinal needle horizontally in the midline but angled slightly towards the head. Some resistance is felt as it passes through the interspinous ligament but, despite what older textbooks say, with modern disposable needles there is no sensation of 'give' as the needle passes through the ligamentum

a line joining the
iliac crests passes
through the level of L4

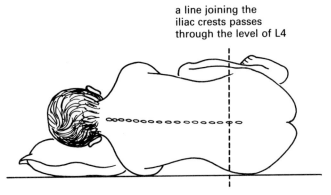

Fig. 11.1   How to position the patient for a lumbar puncture.

flavum and the dura to indicate that the tip of the needle has entered the subarachnoid space. When the tip of the needle is near the dura it is necessary to adopt a technique of advancing the needle a few millimetres at a time, pausing between each advance to withdraw the stylet. If no CSF emerges through the lumen of the needle, replace the stylet and advance the needle a little further.

If, while advancing the needle, you encounter bone, withdraw the needle and reinsert it at a slightly different angle.

Once the tip of the needle is positioned in the subarachnoid space attach the manometer to the hub of the needle using a three-way tap and measure the pressure.

Collect 10 ml of CSF into sterile containers, label them and send them immediately to the laboratory.

Withdraw the needle without replacing the stylet and spray the skin over the puncture with Nobecutane.

Take a sample of venous blood from the patient for estimation of glucose concentration.

ANALYSIS OF CSF

Appearance

Normal CSF is crystal clear. According to the medical convention by which fluids and tissues are described with gastronomic metaphors, the appearance of normal CSF is usually likened to Gordon's gin. When the cell count is raised above a few hundred cells per ml the CSF looks slightly opalescent. In cases of bacterial meningitis there may be many thousands of polymorphonuclear cells per ml and the CSF appears frankly purulent.

CSF following a recent subarachnoid haemorrhage is obviously blood-stained. Red blood cells haemolyse quite quickly in CSF and within a few hours of subarachnoid haemorrhage the CSF takes on a yellow tinge known as *xanthochromia*. This can be seen quite clearly if the specimen is centrifuged.

Sometimes, even with a technically perfect lumbar puncture, the spinal needle punctures a vein lying adjacent to the dura and the CSF obtained is blood-stained. Collecting CSF in three sequential aliquots usually makes it clear that trauma is the reason for the blood-staining because the CSF is clear by the second or third specimen. If any doubt remains, centrifuge a specimen immediately. Xanthochromia of the supernatant indicates that blood was present in the CSF before the lumbar puncture was performed.

Pressure

The normal pressure of CSF is below 20 cm of fluid. If the pressure is unexpectedly very high (that is above 30 cm of fluid) seek neurosurgical advice immediately because of the danger of a pressure cone. Very low pressure either indicates that the needle tip is not properly in the subarachnoid space or that the tip of the needle is abutting a nerve root or that a block is present in the spinal canal. Reinsert the stylet, advance the needle slightly and remeasure the pressure. Do not try to aspirate CSF with a syringe.

Microbiological analysis

CSF is sterile under normal circumstances. Gram stain and culture reveal pyogenic organisms. Ziehl-Nielson stain and culture on Lowenstein-Jensen medium are necessary when tuberculous meningitis is suspected. Special staining and culture techniques are needed to reveal fungal or parasitic infection.

The cell count is normally less than 4 mononuclear cells per ml. A slightly raised cell count (5–50 per ml) may be present in multiple sclerosis or other inflammatory conditions. A greatly raised cell count indicates viral or bacterial infection: in bacterial infection the cells are polymorphs, in viral infection mononuclear cells predominate.

VDRL, TPHA and TPI tests are carried out on CSF in the investigation of neurosyphilis.

Biochemical analysis

Protein concentration is normally between 0.15 and 0.45 g/l and the proportion of γ-globulin is less than 15% of the total. The CSF protein concentration is raised in a number of conditions. A very high protein concentration is typically found in Guillain-Barré syndrome, with an acoustic neuroma and in cases of spinal canal block. Smaller increases in protein concentration occur in many neurological conditions, e.g. intracranial tumour, multiple sclerosis, following cerebral infarction or haemorrhage, neurosyphilis and other inflammatory disorders of the brain and meninges. The CSF protein concentration will, of course, be high if the cell count is raised or if the CSF is contaminated with blood.

The γ-globulin fraction may be raised in multiple sclerosis or any other condition in which intrathecal synthesis of γ-globulin is taking place. Oligoclonal IgG bands should be looked for when multiple sclerosis is suspected; they are present in about 80% of cases, but the finding is not completely specific to this disease.

The glucose concentration in CSF is normally about 60% of the prevailing plasma concentration. In diabetic patients the CSF glucose concentration may be unusually high because of hyperglycaemia. The CSF glucose concentration is abnormally low in bacterial, including tuberculous, meningitis. The interpretation of CSF glucose concentrations is often simplified if the blood glucose concentration at the time of the lumbar puncture was also measured.

Table 11.1   Summary of normal CSF values

Appearance	Crystal clear
Pressure	< 20 cm of fluid
Cell count	< 4 mononuclear cells per ml
Protein concentration	0.15–0.45 g/l
γ-globulin	< 15% of total protein
Oligoclonal IgG bands	Not normally present
Glucose concentration	3.5–6.0 mmol/l

12. Electromyography and nerve conduction studies

The techniques of electromyography and nerve conduction velocity measurement are used in the investigation of diseases of muscle and peripheral nerve. As well as providing confirmation of the clinical diagnosis they are often able to give additional information about the nature of the disease process. Both techniques are safe and though they involve a little discomfort for the patient they are usually easily tolerated.

ELECTROMYOGRAPHY (EMG)

A concentric needle electrode with a diameter of 0.3–0.5 mm is inserted through the skin into the belly of the muscle. The potential difference between the outer and inner electrode is, after suitable amplification, displayed on an oscilloscope screen and simultaneously made audible by connection to a loudspeaker. The electrode picks up electrical muscle activity within a radius of 1–2 mm of its tip, which means that it samples from about 30 motor units.

The electrical activity of the muscle is studied with the muscle fully relaxed, with the muscle undergoing minimal voluntary contraction and with the muscle contracting maximally.

Normal muscle

A normal muscle is electrically silent at rest. When a minimal voluntary contraction is made monophasic, biphasic or triphasic potentials become visible on the screen and are heard as crackles from the loudspeaker. Each potential represents the activity of a single motor unit, i.e. a lower motor neurone and all the muscle fibres innervated by it. The amplitude of these potentials is between 0.5 and 2 mV and their duration is between 4 and 8 ms. With a more powerful voluntary contraction the number of motor units being recruited increases and the individual potentials become superimposed on one another. This appearance is known as an interference pattern.

Denervated muscle

Fibrillations and fasciculations occur spontaneously in denervated muscle. The former represent the spontaneous contraction of a single muscle fibre showing on the screen as a short duration (1−2 ms) potential of about 0.5 mv amplitude and are just audible on the loudspeaker. Fasciculations represent the spontaneous firing of a whole motor unit and look and sound just like the motor units of normal muscle. The presence of fasciculations usually indicates a disease process affecting the anterior horn cell.

Complete denervation abolishes all voluntary contraction of the muscle and no potentials can be detected. Partial denervation results in a reduced interference pattern because of the reduced number of motor units that are available for recruitment. When denervation is chronic, as occurs in diseases that are slowly progressive, the remaining nerve fibres attempt to compensate by increasing the number of colateral terminal branches. Sprouts grow out from the terminals of healthy motor neurones and attempt to reinnervate denervated muscle fibres. This process of reinnervation effectively increases the size of the motor unit so that the size of the electrical potential recorded when the unit fires is larger than normal. Giant potentials, as they are called, are characteristic of the EMG in cases of motor neurone disease.

Myopathy

In myopathic conditions the individual muscle fibres which make up the motor units tend to fire less synchronously than normal. This results in potentials of abnormally low amplitude and of abnormally long duration. The waveform is polyphasic. Spontaneous activity, detectable as a fibrillation, may be present if part of a muscle fibre is functionally denervated by being separated from its endplate region by a necrotic segment. Fasciculations do not occur.

Some muscle diseases, notably dystrophia myotonica, show characteristic electrical abnormalities. Myotonia is due to a membrane abnormality that causes repetitive firing of the muscle fibre. During electromyography this can be heard on the loudspeaker as a noise that is often described as a 'dive-bomber potential'.

The appearance of the EMG in both healthy and diseased muscle is illustrated in Figure 12.1.

NERVE CONDUCTION STUDIES

Motor nerves

A motor nerve can be stimulated percutaneously by applying a DC shock through bipolar electrodes at a point where the nerve runs superficially. If a pair of recording electrodes is placed over a distal muscle served by this nerve the potential of the evoked muscle contraction may be displayed on an oscilloscope screen. By arranging for the oscilloscope sweep to be triggered at the same time as the stimulating shock is delivered it is simple to measure the latency between the stimulus and the muscle contraction. This latency is made up of the conduction time in the peripheral nerve, the time for chemical transmission at the neuromuscular junction and the time taken for the muscle action potential to be generated. If the same nerve is stimulated again at a more distal point and the latency for the muscle action potential again measured, the conduction time over the segment of peripheral nerve between the two points of stimulation can be taken as the difference between the two latencies, since the time taken for neuromuscular transmission and generation of the action potential is the same regardless of where the nerve was stimulated. Assuming that the nerve travels directly between the two stimulation points the distance between them can be estimated with the help of a tape-measure. Knowing both the nerve conduction time and the distance between the two points of stimulation it is simple to calculate a figure for the conduction velocity in the nerve. The method of measurement of motor nerve conduction velocity is illustrated in Figure 12.2.

Sensory nerves

The principle behind the estimation of conduction velocity in a sensory nerve is easier to understand but, because the size of the sensory nerve action potential is small compared with a compound muscle action potential, the measurement is technically more dif-

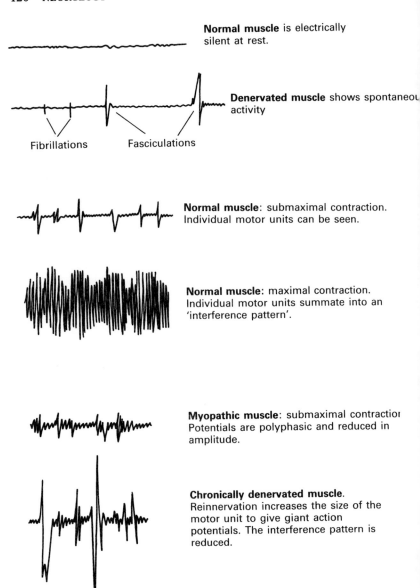

Normal muscle is electrically silent at rest.

Denervated muscle shows spontaneou activity

Fibrillations   Fasciculations

Normal muscle: submaximal contraction. Individual motor units can be seen.

Normal muscle: maximal contraction. Individual motor units summate into an 'interference pattern'.

Myopathic muscle: submaximal contractior Potentials are polyphasic and reduced in amplitude.

Chronically denervated muscle. Reinnervation increases the size of the motor unit to give giant action potentials. The interference pattern is reduced.

Fig. 12.1 Appearances of the EMG in normal and diseased muscle.

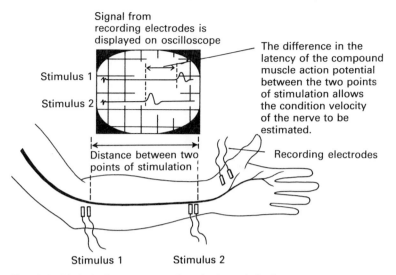

Fig. 12.2   Method of measurement of conduction velocity in a motor nerve.

ficult to carry out. Use of an electronic averaging technique, similar to that described in the section on measurement of cortical evoked potentials, is usually necessary to reduce background noise and clarify the nerve action potential. The nerve is stimulated peripherally and the action potential detected by recording electrodes positioned directly over the nerve. The arrangement is shown in Figure 12.3. The latency is measured from the oscilloscope screen and the distance between the stimulating and recording electrodes measured with a tape measure. The conduction velocity can be calculated directly.

Interpretation of nerve conduction velocity measurements

The compound action potential, whether of nerve or muscle, starts when impulses arrive in the fastest conducting nerve fibres. Nerve conduction velocity measurements indicate therefore, the function of the largest myelinated fibres in the peripheral nerve. No information can be obtained by the techniques described here about the function of the smaller myelinated and non-myelinated fibres.

Remembering that the conclusions apply only to the larger myelinated fibres, interpretation of the results is fairly straightforward. Severe slowing of the conduction velocity, from

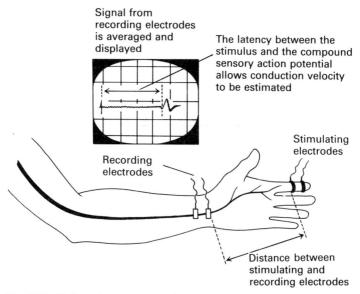

Signal from recording electrodes is averaged and displayed

The latency between the stimulus and the compound sensory action potential allows conduction velocity to be estimated

Stimulating electrodes

Recording electrodes

Distance between stimulating and recording electrodes

Fig. 12.3 Method of measurement of conduction velocity in a sensory nerve.

a normal value of around 60 m/s to less than 35 m/s, indicates a demyelinating process. Slight slowing, to between 50 and 40 m/s, in combination with a reduced amplitude of the evoked action potential, is characteristic of disease affecting the nerve axons. Complete failure to record an action potential following electrical stimulation of the nerve implies that the number of functioning axons within the nerve is severely reduced but no inference can be drawn about the nature of the pathological process involved.

13. The electroencephalogram and evoked responses

The electroencephalogram (EEG) a recording of spontaneous electrical potentials originating in the cerebral cortex, from electrodes fixed to the scalp. These potentials are thought to arise mainly in the apical dendrites of large pyramidal cells in the superficial layers of the cortex. The electrodes used for recording the EEG are large relative to the size of a neurone and are placed some distance away from the cortex with layers of skin, scalp, bone and dura interposed. The EEG is therefore an average of the electrical potentials generated by many thousands of nerve cells.

Evoked responses are the electrical potentials produced in the central nervous system in response to a repeated sensory stimulus. They are generated in the fibre tracts of the spinal cord, structures in the brain stem and in the cerebral cortex and, like the EEG, can be recorded from surface electrodes.

Both the EEG and measurement of evoked responses have the enormous advantage that they are free of risk for the patient. Unfortunately, they are technically quite difficult to perform and the interpretation of the results requires considerable skill and experience. You need not aspire to becoming an expert in the techniques, but you should appreciate how they are carried out and the clinical circumstances in which they are valuable so that you can make the best use of them.

ELECTROENCEPHALOGRAPHY

Electrodes fixed to the scalp in standardized positions allow the attenuated electrical potentials of the underlying cortex to be recorded. A large degree of amplification is necessary and the signal must be filtered to exclude the many sources of artefact. The signals are displayed on the moving paper trace of an 8- or 16-channel pen recorder. The EEG is usually recorded for about 20 minutes; initially the recording is made with the patient lying or sitting quietly, then the patient is asked to hyperventilate and finally there is a period of recording with a flickering strobe light source placed in front of the patient's eyes. These two latter manoeuvres are intended to accentuate epileptic abnormalities.

Some centres have facilities for carrying out prolonged ambulatory EEG monitoring. A small tape-recorder, which can be carried by the patient on his belt, is used to collect the signals from a limited number of scalp electrodes. This technique improves the chances of recording a paroxysmal abnormality.

The normal EEG

In normal adults an 8–13 Hz rhythm, the *alpha rhythm*, predominates. This rhythm is most conspicuous from the posterior electrodes while the patient is relaxed with his eyes closed. In most people the alpha rhythm disappears when the eyes are open. A faster *beta rhythm* (>13 Hz) is also present, especially in the recordings from anteriorly placed electrodes, which is not affected by eye opening and closure.

Two slower rhythms, *theta* (4–8 Hz) and *delta* (<4 Hz), are found in children and adolescents, but are not normally present in adults.

The abnormal EEG

Two main types of abnormality are found on the EEG: epileptic activity and slow wave activity. Epileptic activity shows up on the recording as spikes, sharp waves or a combination of spike and slow wave activity. Unless prolonged EEG monitoring has been carried out, it is rare to capture an actual seizure.

Generalized slow wave activity is usually an indication of a generalized abnormality of brain function, such as may be found in encephalitis, encephalopathy or degenerative neurological disease. Continuous slow waves in a focal distribution suggest the presence of a structural lesion in or just below the cerebral cortex.

Interpretation of the EEG

As a diagnostic test the EEG is neither very specific nor very sensitive. Specificity is poor because different neurological diseases may give rise to similar EEG abnormalities and, perhaps more importantly, because minor EEG 'abnormalities' may be found in individuals without any neurological disease at all. The low sensitivity means that the EEG may be normal in patients with definite neurological disease. When using the results of an EEG to plan the management of a patient, it is essential to bear its limitations in mind.

The EEG is most useful in the investigation of epilepsy. Within the limits discussed above, it may help confirm the clinical diagnosis. Of greater value is its ability to determine the type of epilepsy and to localize the site of an epileptic focus.

EVOKED POTENTIAL STUDIES

When afferent impulses from a stimulated sensory organ reach the cerebral cortex a very small electrical potential is evoked. This potential is normally too small to be recorded but, if the stimulation is repeated many times and the cortical response is electronically averaged, the signal to noise ratio can be improved. The process works like this. The recording from the cortex consists of a minute evoked potential hidden in random background noise. When several hundred recordings are averaged, the background noise is reduced because a random positive deflection in one recording tends to be cancelled out by a random negative deflection in another. The evoked potential by contrast is not random; it occurs at the same point relative to the stimulus on each recording and averaging clarifies rather than diminishes it. Electronic averaging makes it possible to record cortical potentials evoked by visual, auditory and somatosensory stimulation.

Visual evoked potentials (VEP)

An alternating checkerboard pattern in which the black squares change to white and the white squares change to black at a frequency of one change per second is used to provide the visual stimulus. The patient sits quietly looking at the screen on which the stimulus is displayed. Scalp electrodes placed over the occiput pick up the evoked potential which is then amplified, averaged and displayed. The waveform of the potential is complex but for diagnostic purposes measurement of the latency of the major positive deflection which, in normal subjects, occurs about 100 ms after the stimulus, has been found to be the most useful.

Measurement of VEP is of most value in the diagnosis of multiple sclerosis. An abnormally delayed potential provides evidence of a lesion somewhere in the visual pathway. Delay in the VEP is not specific for multiple sclerosis but, in cases where the diagnosis is suspected for other reasons, it provides confirmatory evidence.

Brain stem auditory evoked potentials (BAEP)

The stimulus is a click delivered by a loudspeaker into one ear. Recordings are made from an electrode placed at the vertex. The waveform of the BAEP is polyphasic and each peak corresponds to electrical activity at a particular point in the auditory pathway. The first two positive waves are generated in the auditory nerve and the cochlear nuclei, waves three to five are produced by structures in the pons and midbrain and the much longer latency sixth and seventh wave arise in the auditory cortex.

BAEPs are most useful in the diagnosis of acoustic neuromas, brain stem lesions and multiple sclerosis.

Somatosensory evoked potentials (SSEP)

An electrical stimulus is delivered to a peripheral nerve, usually the median nerve in the arm or the posterior tibial nerve in the leg. Recording electrodes are placed on the scalp overlying the parietal cortex, on the skin over the cervical spinal cord and at Erb's point in the supraclavicular fossa to detect potentials in the brachial plexus.

SSEPs are used in the diagnosis of multiple sclerosis, tumours of the spinal cord and brain stem, and in the investigation of lesions of the brachial plexus.

14. Radiological investigation

Advances in radiological techniques over the past 15 years, with the invention of computerized tomography, digital subtraction angiography and, most recently, magnetic resonance imaging, have revolutionized the practice of neurology. Because these investigations can be performed with very little risk or discomfort they can be used to confirm or exclude the presence of a structural intracranial lesion, even when the degree of clinical suspicion that the patient has such a lesion is low. However, neuroradiological investigations should never be used as a substitute for inadequate clinical skills. When a request is made for a radiological examination the radiologist will wish to know precisely what problem the investigation is intended to solve and how the information gained from the examination is going to affect the management of the patient.

SKULL X-RAY

Plain radiographs demonstrate the bones of the skull but they cannot visualize the relatively radiolucent brain within it. Since CT scanning has become widely available, the main value of skull X-rays has been in the investigation of head injuries to identify skull fracture. However, some intracranial lesions calcify or cause changes in bone and these features may be helpful pointers to the underlying pathology. Several different X-ray projections are needed for a full radiological examination of the skull. The most important are the lateral and antero-posterior views. An antero-posterior view, taken with the brow depressed 35°, shows the posterior fossa and foramen magnum, and a projection taken along an axis running from beneath the chin to the vertex of the skull demonstrates the base of the skull. Special views to show the paranasal air sinuses,

127

the orbits and optic foramina, the pituitary fossa and the internal
auditory meati are sometimes taken.

Skull fractures

Skull fractures appear as linear lucencies. They differ from vascular grooves in that they do not branch or taper and, since both
tables of the skull are involved, they are typically more lucent. Fractures of the base of the skull are often difficult to identify but there
may be indirect evidence from the presence of a fluid level in the
sphenoid sinus caused by bleeding associated with the fracture.

Calcification

Intracranial calcification is seen as a region of high opacity on
the X-ray. Table 14.1 provides a list of the commoner causes.

Pineal shift

The pineal is calcified in a high proportion of adults. It is normally a midline structure and can be identified on both lateral and
anteroposterior views. Lateral displacement of the pineal seen on
the anteroposterior film is a sign of a space-occupying lesion in
the contralateral cerebral hemisphere.

Expansion of the pituitary fossa

Tumours of the pituitary gland enlarge the bony outline of the
pituitary fossa. Asymmetrical expansion may be visible as an apparent double floor of the fossa on a lateral skull film.

Raised intracranial pressure

In chronic cases of raised intracranial pressure the posterior clinoid
processes of the pituitary fossa gradually become eroded.

Table 14.1   Causes of intracranial calcification

Physiological	Pathological
Calcification of pineal choroid plexus falx	Craniopharyngioma Oligodendroglioma Meningioma Arteriovenous malformation Toxoplasmosis Hypoparathyroidism

Basilar impression

On a lateral skull X-ray a line drawn from the end of the hard palate to the posterior margin of the foramen magnum normally lies above the cervical spine. If the odontoid peg protrudes above this line a congenital abnormality of the craniovertebral junction should be suspected.

Bony erosions

Multiple small discrete lucencies in the vault of the skull occur in multiple myeloma and in primary hyperparathyroidism. Meningiomas may cause localized erosion of bone, sometimes in association with areas of hyperostosis. Widening of the internal auditory meatus is a typical feature of acoustic neuromas.

Opacification of sinuses

Opacification of the paranasal air sinuses or mastoid air cells is a sign of infection of these structures. In a patient with neurological signs, opacification of the sinuses raises the possibility of a subdural empyema or an intracerebral abscess.

COMPUTERIZED TOMOGRAPHY (CT)

Multiple finely collimated X-ray beams and an array of crystal detectors replace the single X-ray source and radiographic film of conventional X-rays. Computer processing of many thousands of readings from the detectors enables the degree of X-ray absorption for individual small volumes of tissue to be calculated and these data are used to produce high definition images of the structure under examination. The brain is usually visualized as a series of transverse sections each a few millimeters in thickness. Computer reconstruction of the images in a coronal or saggital plane is also possible— a technique that is particularly valuable in the investigation of lesions of the pituitary fossa and the orbit.

Intravenous injection of contrast medium is frequently used to increase the amount of information obtained from the CT scan. Enhancement of a lesion following injection of contrast medium indicates either that the lesion is highly vascular, or that extravasation of contrast medium is taking place because of breakdown of the blood-brain barrier, or that a combination of both effects is present.

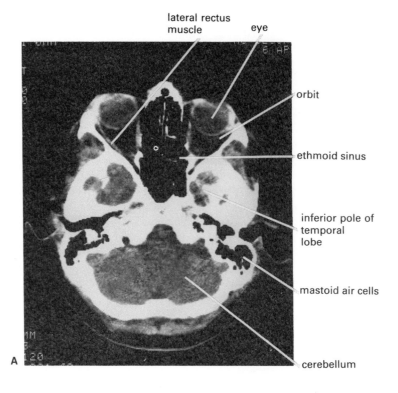

lateral rectus muscle

eye

orbit

ethmoid sinus

inferior pole of temporal lobe

mastoid air cells

cerebellum

A

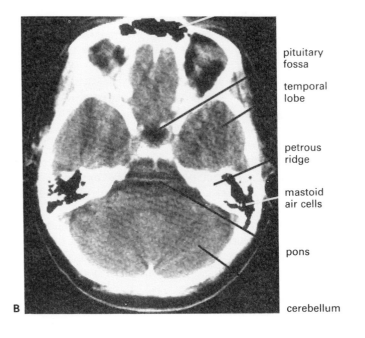

pituitary fossa

temporal lobe

petrous ridge

mastoid air cells

pons

cerebellum

B

frontal sinus

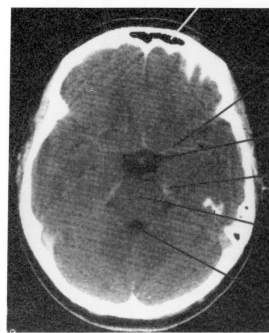

middle cerebral artery

pituitary stalk

posterior cerebral artery

midbrain

quadrigeminal cistern

C

frontal horn of lateral ventricle

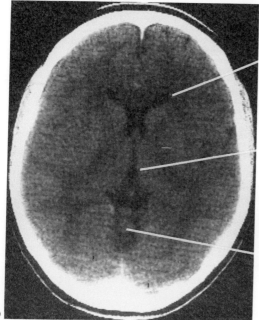

third ventricle

superior vermis

D

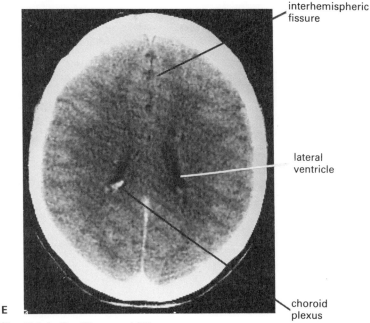

interhemispheric
fissure

lateral
ventricle

E

choroid
plexus

Fig. 14.1 A–E   The normal CT scan.

The normal anatomy of the brain as visualized by CT scan is shown in Figure 14.1. Abnormal features show themselves in four main ways:

1. Abnormal tissue density
2. Mass effect
3. Loss of normal tissue
4. Abnormal pattern of enhancement.

Abnormal tissue density

Tissue density depends on how much attenuation the tissue produces in the X-ray beams transversing it. Tissues with a high degree of attenuation show up on a CT scan at the whiter end of the grey scale; structures of low attenuation show up at the blacker end. Lesions may be identified if they differ from normal brain in the degree of attenuation that they produce. Lesions of lower attenuation than normal brain, and therefore showing darker, are often described as being of low density. Lesions of high attenuation, seen as lighter in colour than normal brain, are described as having high density.

Mass effect

Space-occupying lesions distort the normal tissue around them and are said to show a mass effect. Evidence of mass effect may be visible as a shift in the position of the cerebral ventricles or lateral displacement of the normal midline structures.

Loss of normal tissue

Loss of normal tissue results in areas of decreased attenuation within the substance of the brain. Secondary effects of tissue loss, enlargement of the cerebral ventricles and widening of cerebral sulci, Sylvian and interhemispheric fissures, may also be apparent.

Enhancement

Increased enhancement of tissue following intravenous injection of contrast medium is seen as an increase in tissue density. It indicates a vascular abnormality—either an increase in the amount of blood flow or an increase in the permeability of the vessels to contrast medium.

Different types of lesions have characteristic appearances on CT scan. The appearances of some of the most important are described below.

Cerebral infarction

The CT scan appearances remain normal for the first 12 hours or so after infarction. The earliest signs are due to brain swelling and there is effacement of the cortical sulci overlying the area of infarction and displacement of the ventricular system. The area of infarction itself becomes clearly visible after a few days as a low density region in the distribution of the territory of the occluded vessel. Both grey and white matter are affected as distinct from tumours and infective processes in which low density caused by oedema is usually confined to white matter. The appearance of cerebral infarction at this stage is shown in Figure 14.2. Injection of contrast medium is best avoided in the acute phase as it may lead to extension of the zone of infarction but, if given because there is doubt about the diagnosis, striking enhancement may be seen on the periphery of the infarct.

After the acute phase, when brain swelling has resolved, an infarcted area is visible as an area of decreased attenuation. Loss of

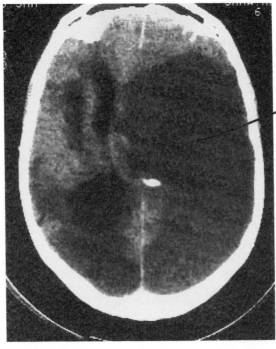

low density
area of
infarction in
territory of
L middle cerebral
artery

Fig. 14.2   Cerebral infarction. Note the massive R to L shift of intracranial structures produced by oedema and low density in both occipital lobes, caused by secondary ischaemia from compression of posterior cerebral arteries.

brain tissue may be indicated by dilatation of the adjacent ventricle and cerebral sulci.

Primary intracerebral haemorrhage

A cerebral haematoma is seen on CT scanning as an area of homogeneous high density surround by a thin rim of low density. If the haematoma also ruptures into the cerebral ventricles high density will be seen within the ventricular system.

Cerebral tumours

Gliomas

Malignant gliomas have irregular margins, enhance irregularly and often contain areas of low density, which represent necrotic areas within the tumours (Fig. 14.3).

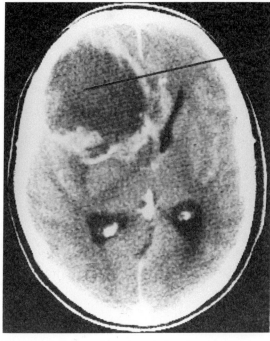

R frontal
glioma

Fig. 14.3 Frontal glioma. Note irregularly enhancing rim, low-density necrotic centre, obliteration of the frontal horn of the R lateral ventricle and displacement of the L lateral ventricle.

Gliomas of low-grade malignancy typically have well-defined margins and are of uniform low density with little or no enhancement following the injection of contrast. Areas of calcification may be present within the tumour. This feature is commonly seen in oligodendrogliomas.

Meningiomas

These tumours arise from the meninges and always have a site of dural attachment. The commonest sites are the convexity of the vault of the skull, often in a parasagittal position and adjacent to the wings of the sphenoid bone, the olfactory grooves and the sella turcica. On a CT scan meningiomas appear as well-defined masses of uniformly high density. They enhance strongly and tend to be surrounded by an area of low density oedema (Fig. 14.4).

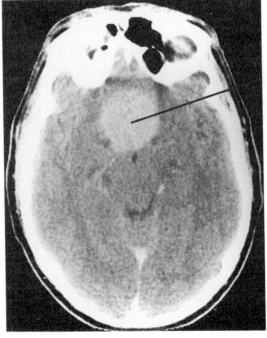

meningioma,
arising from
tuberculum
sellae

Fig. 14.4   Meningioma. Note homogeneous high density with surrounding
rim of low-density oedema.

Metastatic tumour

Metastatic disease provides no diagnostic difficulty if multiple
lesions are visible on the CT scan and a primary tumour is known.
Solitary metastases are harder to diagnose with certainty. Typically they are seen as well-defined high-density areas surrounded
by a rim of low-density oedema. The most common site is at the
junction of grey and white matter. They usually enhance
strongly after the injection of contrast medium. The central part
of the tumour deposit is often necrotic and appears as a
low-density area.

Abscess

Cerebral abscesses appear as circumscribed areas of low density
surrounded by a thin rim of high density, which enhances
strongly after contrast (Fig. 14.5).

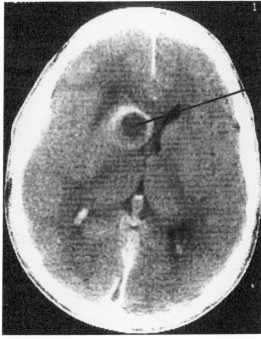

cerebral
abscess

Fig. 14.5 Cerebral abscess. Note round low density area with strongly enhancing rim.

Demyelination

Small low-density areas in a periventricular distribution are characteristic of multiple sclerosis. Sometimes the areas will enhance, particularly if the lesions are the result of a recent exacerbation. Rarely, the area of demyelination is large and can even show a mass effect.

Subarachnoid haemorrhage

Patients who present with sudden onset of occipital headache in whom subarachnoid haemorrhage is suspected require urgent radiological investigation. A CT scan should be arranged as soon as possible as blood in the subarachnoid space becomes less easy to detect with time. If blood is detected on the scan, a lumbar puncture to confirm the diagnosis is unnecessary.

Subarachnoid blood is of high density compared with normal brain. Clues about the origin of the bleeding can be obtained from the distribution of the blood. The presence of blood in the inter-hemispheric fissure or a haematoma in one of the frontal lobes suggests that the source is an aneurysm of the anterior communicating artery. Aneurysms at the bifurcation of the middle cerebral artery often bleed into the Sylvian fissure, whereas aneurysms of the posterior communicating arteries and vertebrobasilar circulation usually bleed into the cisterns that surround the brain stem.

Arteriovenous malformations show up as patches of punctate calcification and serpiginous areas of high density which represent dilated blood vessels.

Trauma

Trauma to the head may, if severe, result in contusion of the brain, haematoma formation, or bleeding into the subarachnoid, subdural or extradural spaces. Intracerebral haematomas appear as uniform areas of high density with a surrounding rim of low density. There is no clear-cut distinction between a haematoma and a contusion. Lesions in which the high-density blood is not homogeneous but interspersed with areas of low density are usually described as contusions. Surgical exploration of such lesions usually reveals an area of softened and damaged brain containing small extravasations of blood, but no large collection which can be drained.

An extradural haematoma appears as a high-density area overlying the cerebral hemisphere with a characteristic biconvex lens shape.

Subdural collections of blood conform to the shape of the cerebral hemisphere, spreading over the surface of the brain and having a concave inner margin. Subdural collections may also be found in the interhemispheric fissure and overlying the tentorium. They tend to increase in size with time, perhaps because of the osmotic effect of lysing red blood cells. The process results in a gradual decrease of the density of the subdural collection and 2−3 weeks after the initial bleed the collection has the same density as the underlying brain. Diagnosis may be difficult if the CT scan is performed at this stage. If the collection is unilateral there will be effacement of the cerebral sulci and evidence of mass effect—displacement of the ventricular system and mid-line structures. The appearance of a unilateral isodense chronic subdural collection is shown in Figure 14.6. A proportion of subdural collections are bilateral and the only signs on CT scanning may be compression

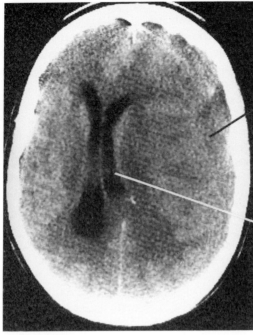

isodense
subdural
collection

compression
of lateral
ventricles
and shift
of midline

Fig. 14.6 Chronic subdural haematoma.

of the ventricles and effacement of cerebral sulci. Intravenous contrast may be helpful in these cases as the brain will enhance but the haematoma will not.

MAGNETIC RESONANCE IMAGING

This technique makes use of the behaviour of protons in a strong magnetic field. Being electrically charged, protons orientate themselves along lines of magnetic force. A brief radiofrequency electromagnetic pulse momentarily perturbs their alignment. As they return to their former position the protons act as tiny magnets and their position can be detected by the electromagnetic forces that they induce in a surrounding coil. Computerized imaging methods can then be employed to construct maps of proton density in the substance being examined. In living material the vast majority of protons are found in the hydrogen atoms of water and these maps reflect differences in the water content of the various tissues.

This technique is of great potential value in the investigation of disorders of the brain and spinal cord and has several advantages over CT scanning. The lack of artefact from bone allows clear images of structures in the posterior fossa, at the base of the brain and in the vertebral canal to be obtained. In the investigation of lesions of temporal lobes, cerebellum, brainstem and cervical spinal cord magnetic resonance imaging is superior to CT scanning. Magnetic resonance imaging is also better than conventional CT in distinguishing grey from white matter and is therefore a more sensitive way of detecting plaques of demyelination. There is the further advantage that patients examined by magnetic resonance techniques are not exposed to any ionizing radiation.

ANGIOGRAPHY

The technique of angiography involves the injection of a bolus of contrast medium at high pressure into an artery and taking a series of X-rays in rapid succession in order to capture the arterial, capillary and venous phases of the progress of the contrast medium through the vasculature. For cerebral angiography, contrast medium is introduced either by direct puncture of a carotid or vertebral artery or, more usually, by introducing a flexible catheter into the femoral artery and then manoeuvring it so that the tip lies in the origin of the carotid or vertebral arteries in the arch of the aorta. The arterial phase of a normal carotid angiogram is shown in Figure 14.7.

The recent development of digital subtraction angiography, a computer technique in which the image of the background structures is digitized, recorded and removed from the final radiograph, improves the contrast of the angiogram and allows the examination to be carried out with much smaller volumes of contrast medium.

The main uses of cerebral angiography are in the investigation of subarachnoid haemorrhage, cerebral tumours and cerebrovascular disease.

Cerebral angiography is needed in cases of subarachnoid haemorrhage in order to identify the site of bleeding and to determine the type of vascular abnormality which has led to the rupture of the vessel — usually either an aneurysm or an arteriovenous malformation. An aneurysm appears as a focal dilatation of an artery, often occurring at a site of arterial bifurcation. Several different radiographic projections are used to establish the direction

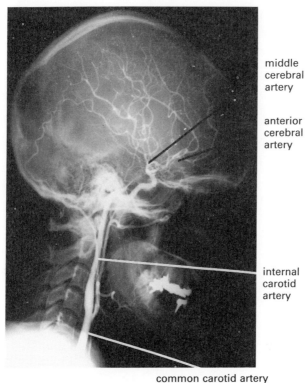

middle
cerebral
artery

anterior
cerebral
artery

internal
carotid
artery

common carotid artery

Fig. 14.7   Normal carotid angiogram (lateral view).

in which the aneurysm is pointing, its size, the position of the neck of the aneurysm and any irregularities in its shape. Figure 14.8 shows the angiographic appearance of an aneurysm of the middle cerebral artery.

In cases of subarachnoid haemorrhage from arteriovenous malformation, knowledge of the blood supply and venous drainage as well as its site and size are important in order to decide whether surgical intervention is possible. The arteries that supply the arteriovenous malformation are dilated and tortuous. They fill with contrast more quickly than normal vessels. The malformation itself appears as a tangle of dilated vessels. The draining veins fill early and are also dilated.

Angiography may also be valuable in the diagnosis of intracranial tumours and in planning the surgical approach. The tumour may be delineated either by an abnormal tumour circu-

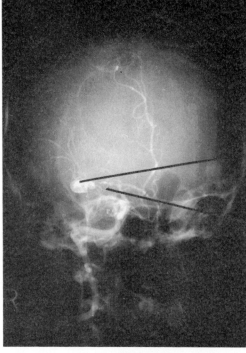

aneurysm

spasm of
middle cerebral
artery

Fig. 14.8   Right carotid angiogram showing aneurysm of middle cerebral
artery (Oblique view).

lation or by the effect it has on displacing normal vessels from
their usual position.

Where surgical intervention (e.g. carotid endarterectomy) is
being considered for the treatment of occlusive cerebrovascular
disease, angiography is needed preoperatively to identify the site
and severity of the arterial stenosis and to evaluate the condition
of the rest of the cerebral vasculature.

Angiographic procedures are not without risk and should only
be carried out when the results are likely to affect the management of the patient. After subarachnoid haemorrhage there is a
considerable danger that angiography will provoke arterial spasm
(see Fig. 14.8) which may lead to ischaemia and deterioration in
the patient's condition. The risk of spasm is greatest in patients
whose initial clinical state is poor and most neurosurgeons will
reserve angiography for patients without focal neurological deficit

or depression in conscious level. Less common complications of angiography include embolization from the tip of the catheter, local damage to the artery at the site of puncture and allergic reactions to the injected contrast medium.

X-RAYS OF THE SPINE AND MYELOGRAPHY

Plain X-ray films of the spine will reveal fractures, dislocations or vertebral subluxation and are essential investigations in cases of spinal trauma. In some cases of non-traumatic spinal cord or root compression bony changes may provide information about underlying pathology. Erosion of the pedicle of the vertebral arch or collapse of a vertebral body is suggestive of a secondary tumour deposit. Evidence of degenerative disc disease may be seen on a lateral film as narrowing of the disc space and hypertrophy of the facet joints. However, for a definite diagnosis it is almost always necessary to procede to myelography.

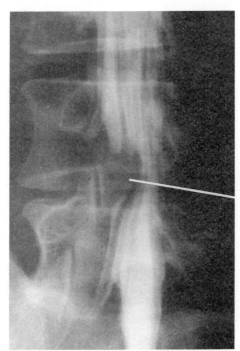

prolapsed disc indents column of contrast medium and obliterates the fifth lumbar root pocket.

Fig. 14.9   Prolapse of lumbar intervertebral disc.

Myelography

The injection of water-soluble contrast medium into the sub-arachnoid space allows the spinal cord and nerve roots to be visual-ized on X-ray. The contrast medium is introduced by lumbar puncture or by lateral cervical puncture and the flow of contrast medium along the spinal canal can be controlled by tilting the table on which the patient is lying.

Obstruction to the free passage of contrast medium along the spinal canal indicates the site of compression and may show whether the lesion is extradural, intradural or intramedullary. CT scanning of a segment of the vertebral column, once the site of the lesion has been accurately located, may allow the nature and ex-tent of the lesion to be defined more precisely.

A more limited examination, known as *radiculography*, in which the contrast medium introduced by lumbar puncture is restricted to the lower end of the spinal canal, is frequently used in the in-vestigation of suspected intervertebral disc prolapse. Figure 14.9 shows the appearance of lumbar nerve root compression by a lateral prolapse of the L4/5 intervertebral disc.

Disorders of the nervous system

15. Cerebrovascular disease

Cerebrovascular disease is a major cause of death and disability in China, Japan and all countries in the Western world. All doctors are bound to encounter many cases and it is essential to understand both the manifestations of the disease and the underlying factors which predispose to it.

In order to clarify one's thoughts about a patient with a suspected stroke two separate but related questions have to be answered. The first is: what is the pathological mechanism by which the patient's cerebral blood flow has been compromised? This question usually resolves itself into deciding whether the stroke was caused by occlusion of a cerebral artery by thrombosis or embolism, or whether it was due to haemorrhage into the substance of the brain or into the subarachnoid space following the rupture of a vessel.

The second question is: can this patient's clinical picture be understood in terms of the anatomy of the cerebral blood vessels? Put more simply, this means which blood vessel do you think is involved? If the patient's signs and symptoms cannot be explained by an area of ischaemia that corresponds to the territory of a cerebral artery, a diagnosis of stroke must not be accepted without further investigation. Cerebrovascular disease is so common that there is a tendency to accept a diagnosis of stroke uncritically in any elderly patient admitted with signs and symptoms that are vaguely neurological. Many patients with a depressed conscious level due to hypothermia, or drug overdose, or diabetic coma have been labelled as 'stroke' at the time of admission and had the correct diagnosis established only after unnecessary delay.

This chapter discusses these two questions in turn.

PATHOLOGY

Thrombosis

Atheromatous plaques in large arteries and arteriosclerotic disease of smaller vessels disturb laminar blood flow and predispose to thrombus formation. Thrombus may occlude a vessel either at the site where it is formed or may become detached and cause embolic occlusion distally. Risk factors for the development of atheroma in cerebral vessels are similar to the well-known risk factors for coronary artery disease. Hypertension, cigarette smoking and diabetes are clearly implicated, but hyperlipidaemia may be less important in cerebral than in coronary artery disease.

A less common underlying cause of cerebral thrombosis is the presence of inflammation of the arterial wall. Thrombosis of cerebral arteries may be a complication of vasculitis associated with collagen-vascular diseases such as systemic lupus erythematosus and polyarteritis.

Disorders of blood which lead to a hypercoagulable state, e.g. polycythaemia, idiopathic and thrombocytopenic purpura, thrombocythaemia and other coagulopathies, also predispose to thrombosis of cerebral vessels.

Embolism

Cardiac disease, especially if disease of the mitral valve or atrial fibrillation is present, may lead to embolus formation. The following list includes the most important cardiac conditions that give rise to emboli:

1. Rheumatic heart disease
2. Infective endocarditis
3. Prosthetic heart valves
4. Ventricular aneurysm
5. Recent myocardial infarction
6. Atrial myxoma.

Atheromatous plaques in the arch of the aorta or in the carotid arteries (the bifurcation of the internal and external carotid arteries in the neck is a very frequent site of plaque formation) are also common sources of cerebral emboli.

Haemorrhage

Intracerebral haemorrhage and subarachnoid haemorrhage result from the rupture of an intracranial artery. The underlying cause is a defect in the wall of the artery, either at a site of aneurysmal dilatation or at an arteriovenous malformation.

Aneurysms of the cerebral circulation are of two types. Small sacular aneurysms, known as berry aneurysms because of their size and shape, are found on the circle of Willis and its major branches, usually at a point of arterial bifurcation. The cause of these aneurysms is not fully understood but there is evidence that they develop as a result of a local congenital defect in the structure of the arterial wall. The second type of aneurysm is found on the smaller perforating vessels which supply the deep structures of the brain. They are microaneurysms, 1–2 mm in diameter, and are often multiple. Systemic hypertension is a strong predisposing factor in their development.

Arteriovenous malformations are developmental abnormalities of cerebral vasculature. They consist of a tortuous mass of vessels in which there is direct shunting of arterial blood into dilated veins. They may enlarge slowly but are not truly neoplastic. Although most frequently found within the cerebral hemispheres they also occur in the posterior fossa and in the vasculature of the spinal cord.

ANATOMY OF THE CEREBRAL CIRCULATION

Four major vessels arising from the arch of the aorta, two carotid arteries and two vertebral arteries, supply the brain with blood. At the base of the brain these vessels communicate by anastomotic channels—the circle of Willis—which can, to an extent that varies between individuals, compensate for decreased blood flow in one of these vessels. On each side of the brain three arteries, the anterior, middle and posterior cerebral arteries, arise from the circle of Willis to supply the cerebral hemispheres. Figure 15.1 shows the arterial supply to the brain.

The anterior cerebral artery

This artery is a branch of the internal carotid artery and supplies blood to the medial surface of the hemispheres. Don't make the common mistake of assuming from its name that it supplies the frontal lobes.

The middle cerebral artery

This artery is effectively a direct continuation of the internal

The circle of Willis

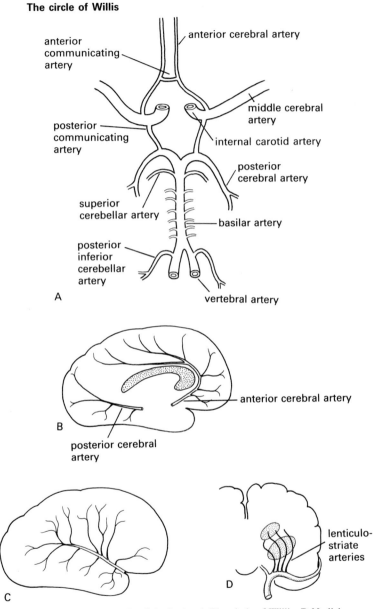

Fig. 15.1 The arterial supply of the brain. **A** The circle of Willis. **B** Medial surface of hemisphere showing anterior and posterior cerebral arteries. **C** Lateral surface of hemisphere showing area supplied by middle cerebral artery. **D** Perforating lenticulostriate arteries arising from the proximal segment of the middle cerebral artery. These arteries supply the internal capsule, the thalamus and the basal ganglia.

carotid artery; it supplies almost the whole of the lateral surface of the hemisphere and gives off deep perforating branches to the internal capsule and the basal ganglia.

The posterior cerebral artery

The posterior cerebral artery, formed from and mainly fed by the basilar artery, supplies the occipital lobe and also the undersurface of the temporal lobe.

The vertebrobasilar arterial system

The brain stem and the cerebellum are supplied by branches of the vertebral and basilar arteries.

SYNDROMES OF THE CEREBRAL ARTERIES

Anterior cerebral artery

Occlusion of the anterior cerebral artery proximal to the anterior communicating artery is symptomless, because blood flow can be maintained from the contralateral anterior cerebral artery. Occlusion of the artery distal to the anterior communicating artery deprives the medial surface of the hemisphere of its blood supply and results in weakness and sensory loss in the contralateral leg. Refer to Figure 2.2 on page 10 for a reminder that the cortical representation of the leg in the motor cortex is on the medial surface of the hemisphere. The superomedial part of the frontal lobe which contains the cortical centre for bladder control is adjacent to the area of motor cortex in which the leg is represented and anterior cerebral artery occlusion sometimes causes urinary incontinence too.

Middle cerebral artery

A complete proximal occlusion of the middle cerebral artery causes infarction of a large area of cortex on the lateral surface of the hemisphere. The clinical picture is of a contralateral hemiparesis in which, typically, the arm is more severely affected than the leg. In addition there is a contralateral sensory loss (hemianaesthesia), a contralateral homonymous hemianopia (because the optic radiation is affected), aphasia if the infarct is in the dominant hemisphere and signs of parietal lobe dysfunction, particularly if the infarct is in the non-dominant hemisphere.

The large volume of infarcted brain that results from complete proximal occlusion of the middle cerebral artery is accompanied by considerable oedema and swelling. The swelling may compress and distort other brain structures and cause further neurological damage. The patient's conscious level is often depressed and there may be signs in the limbs ipsilateral to the occluded artery because of compression of the opposite cerebral peduncle.

Occlusion of one of the distal branches of the middle cerebral artery causes a more limited neurological syndrome. The clinical features depend on which branch is occluded. Occlusion of an anterior branch results in hemiparesis and, in the dominant hemisphere, expressive dysphasia. Occlusion of a posterior branch causes a cortical type of sensory loss, a predominantly receptive dysphasia if the dominant hemisphere is affected and parietal lobe dysfunction.

A number of small lenticulostriate arteries arise from the middle cerebral artery near its origin. These vessels perforate the substance of the brain to supply the basal ganglia and the internal capsule. Although the amount of brain supplied by any of these vessels individually, is small, occlusion is likely to result in hemiparesis because the whole of the motor outflow from the cortex is concentrated in the internal capsule. Syndromes caused by occlusion of small perforating vessels are discussed later in this section under the heading of lacunar infarction.

Posterior cerebral artery

Proximal occlusion of this vessel causes infarction of the occipital lobe and results in a contralateral homonymous hemianopia. Small perforating vessels arising from the proximal part of the posterior cerebral artery supply the posterior thalamus. Occlusion of these vessels causes thalamic infarction, which results in a hemisensory disturbance affecting the whole of the contralateral side of the body. If the subthalamic nucleus is infarcted hemiballismus may result.

Internal carotid artery

The clinical features of internal carotid artery occlusion are variable and depend on the extent to which the anastomoses of the circle of Willis can compensate. The largest branch of the internal carotid artery is the middle cerebral artery and occlusion of the internal carotid artery may not be distinguishable clinically from a proximal occlusion of the middle cerebral artery. At the other end of the clinical spectrum, complete occlusion of the internal carotid artery can occur without causing any symptoms at all.

Basilar artery occlusion

Proximal occlusion of the basilar artery is often fatal because the whole brain stem is made ischaemic. Distal occlusion, where the artery bifurcates to form the posterior cerebral arteries, results in bilateral infarction of both occipital lobes and causes cortical blindness. The pupillary response to light is preserved. One amazing feature of cortical blindness due to basilar artery occlusion is that the patient denies his disability; it seems that he has not only lost the ability to see, but also the ability to think in visual terms at all.

Occlusion of branches of the basilar artery that supply the brain stem cause a variety of syndromes depending on the precise site of infarction. Many of these syndromes have eponymous names, but since most are rare, at least in their pure form, there is little to be gained by memorizing the details. Because of the close anatomical relationship of descending and ascending fibre pathways, cranial nerve nuclei and cerebellar connections, infarction within the brain stem is characterized by combinations of cranial nerve lesions, limb signs, nystagmus and dysarthria.

Vertebral artery occlusion

Occlusion of a vertebral artery may result in infarction of the lateral part of the lower medulla in the territory of the posterior inferior cerebellar artery. Each posterior inferior cerebellar artery arises from a vertebral artery immediately proximal to the point where the vertebral arteries join to form the basilar artery. It is the only vessel supplied exclusively by a single vertebral artery and its area of distribution is therefore most vulnerable to ischaemia following occlusion of a vertebral artery.

Lateral medullary infarction is by far the commonest of the brain stem vascular syndromes. The affected area is shown in Figure 15.2. Ischaemia of the inferior cerebellar peduncle and

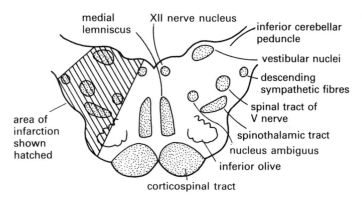

Fig. 15.2 The area of medullary infarction resulting from occlusion of the posterior inferior cerebellar artery.

cerebellar hemisphere causes ipsilateral ataxia of limbs, nystagmus and dysarthria. Within the medulla the descending sympathetic fibres, the spinal tract of the 5th cranial nerve and the nucleus ambiguus are affected causing, respectively, an ipsilateral Horner's syndrome, ipsilateral sensory loss over the face and paralysis of the ipsilateral muscles of the pharynx and larynx. The ascending fibres of the spinothalamic tract are also involved; this causes loss of sensation, pain and temperature over the contralateral side of the body. Note the *crossed* sensory loss caused by a lateral medullary lesion; sensory loss on the face is ipsilateral while that on the body is contralateral.

Lacunar infarction

Blood is supplied to the deep structures of the cerebral hemispheres and brainstem by numerous small perforating arteries arising from the proximal segments of the middle and posterior cerebral arteries and from the basilar artery. Occlusion of one of these vessels causes a small area of infarction—a lacune. Several specific syndromes are known to be the result of lacunar infarction.

A pure motor stroke involving face, arm and leg, or sometimes just the face and arm, or just the arm and leg, indicates a small infarct in the posterior limb of the internal capsule of the contralateral hemisphere.

A pure sensory stroke, again involving at least two out of face, arm and leg, indicates a small infarct in the posterior part of the thalamus.

A syndrome of ataxic hemiparesis with features of ipsilateral cerebellar and corticospinal tract dysfunction occurs with small infarcts in the pons. The cerebellar and corticospinal features may be quite localized. One manifestation is the *dysarthria-clumsy hand syndrome* in which, as you would expect from the name, there is dysarthria, weakness and ataxia of the ipsilateral hand and sometimes facial weakness in addition.

Many solitary lacunar infarcts are silent, but multiple lacunar infarction may result in a syndrome of progressive dementia (see Chap. 20). The dementia is often accompanied by a shuffling gait, sometimes called *marché à petits pas*, and features of a pseudobulbar palsy.

TRANSIENT ISCHAEMIC ATTACKS

Transient ischaemic attacks (TIAs) are defined as episodes of focal neurological disturbance caused by cerebrovascular disease in which symptoms persist for less than 24 hours. To make a diagnosis of a TIA it is essential to exclude, usually by taking a careful history, other disorders which cause transient neurological disturbance, such as partial epilepsy, migraine, cardia arrythmia, hypoglycaemia and hyperventilation.

TIAs are important because they may be a warning sign of a stroke—a permanent ischaemic attack. Between 5% and 10% of patients who experience a TIA will develop a stroke within the 12 months following the attack.

The most likely mechanism for the pathogenesis of TIAs is that platelet emboli, formed on atherosclerotic plaques in the large extracranial vessels, are carried distally and temporarily occlude distal branches of the cerebral circulation before breaking up and dispersing. An alternative mechanism is that, because of a fall in cardiac output, perhaps as a result of a cardiac dysrhythmia, the flow in a stenosed artery becomes critically reduced leading to symptoms of ischaemia in the area of brain supplied by that vessel.

Amaurosis fugax

This is a particular form of TIA in which there is a transient loss of vision in one eye lasting a few minutes to a few hours. The cause is a transient occlusion of the ophthalmic artery usually from an embolus which has formed on a plaque of atheroma in the carotid artery, but occasionally from an embolic source in the heart.

Careful ophthalmoscopy during or after an attack of amaurosis fugax sometimes reveals small emboli in the retinal arteries. Amaurosis fugax carries the same significance for investigation and management as a transient ischaemic attack, which indeed is what it is.

TIAs in the distribution of other arteries

TIAs which result from transient obstruction in the territory of a carotid artery cause symptoms similar to those of middle cerebral artery occlusion: hemiparesis, sensory disturbance over one half of the body or dysphasia. If the TIA is in the vertebrobasilar distribution there are symptoms of brain stem dysfunction such as vertigo, diplopia and loss of consciousness. Rarely, if the circulation in the posterior cerebral arteries is affected, transient cortical blindness can occur.

INVESTIGATION OF STROKE AND TRANSIENT ISCHAEMIC ATTACKS

The diagnosis of stroke or TIA can usually be made from the clinical evidence. If there is any doubt, a CT brain scan should be performed. This will allow alternative diagnoses to be excluded and, in cases of completed stroke, demonstrate the area of infarction. If the clinical diagnosis is of embolic stroke and anticoagulation is being considered, a CT brain scan is necessary before treatment is started to ensure that no intracerebral haemorrhage is present.

TIAs and non-disabling minor strokes require further investigation in order to identify treatable predisposing factors and prevent recurrence. The vigour with which these investigations are pursued will depend on the age and clinical condition of the patient. Investigations which may be appropriate are given in Table 15.1.

TREATMENT OF STROKE AND TRANSIENT ISCHAEMIC ATTACKS

Acute cerebral infarction

A number of specific measures aimed at improving cerebral circulation, reducing oedema, or decreasing cerebral metabolism have

Table 15.1 Investigation of stroke and TIAs

Predisposing factor	Investigation
Haematological	
polycythaemia	Full blood count
thrombocythaemia	Platelet count
sickle cell disease	Peripheral blood film
Diabetes mellitus	Fasting blood glucose
Neurosyphilis	VDRL
Cardiac disease (see list on p. 148)	ECG
	Echocardiography
Vasculitis	
systemic lupus erythematosus	ESR
polyarteritis	ANF
Extracranial carotid artery disease	Non-invasive Doppler imaging
	Angiography

been tried in the treatment of acute cerebral infarction, but, at present, there is no general agreement about their value.

Supportive nursing care, with particular attention to avoiding pressure sores and maintaining adequate hydration, is essential. The patient must be turned regularly and frequently. A nasogastric tube may be necessary if the patient is unable to swallow adequate quantities of fluid. Urinary incontinence may require catheterization or the use of an appliance. Regular chest physiotherapy reduces the chances of chest infection. Physiotherapy for both normal and paralysed limbs prevents joint stiffness and contractures. Active rehabilitation with the help of physiotherapists, occupational therapists and, if language difficulties are present, speech therapists should begin as soon as practicable.

Prevention of recurrence

For minor strokes and TIAs, treatment directed towards the prevention of further ischaemic episodes should be the primary concern. Systemic hypertension must be treated, but care should be taken to avoid any sudden reduction in blood pressure. Polycythaemia, if present, may require venesection and other measures to reduce blood viscosity. All patients should be strongly advised to stop smoking cigarettes. The evidence that aspirin in low dose is of value in the secondary prevention of stroke is now fairly clear. In the absence of active peptic ulcer disease or other contraindications, soluble aspirin in a dose of 300 mg daily should be prescribed. Anticoagulation should be considered for those patients in whom investigations have shown a cardiac source of emboli.

Surgical treatment of an isolated carotid stenosis by endarterectomy is an attractively logical measure but there is, as yet, no evidence from controlled trials that this treatment improves the prognosis for the patient. A large trial is in progress and the results should be available within a year or two. Since the procedure carries a low but significant morbidity and mortality it seems best to reserve angiography and endarterectomy for those patients who are entered into the trial.

PRIMARY INTRACEREBRAL HAEMORRHAGE

Between 10% and 20% of strokes are not the result of thrombosis or embolism, but are due to rupture of a blood vessel and haemorrhage into the substance of the brain. Haemorrhage usually occurs from small perforating vessels whose walls have been affected by chronic systemic hypertension Loss of smooth muscle and elastic tissue results in the formation of small dilatations and aneurysms. These are weak points in the arteries and liable to rupture. A proportion of intracerebral haemorrhages, especially in younger patients, arise from developmental defects in cerebral vasculature—arteriovenous malformations. The majority of intracerebral haemorrhages occur in regions of the brain richly supplied with small perforating arteries: the region of the basal ganglia, the pons and the cerebellum.

The outlook depends very much on the size of the haemorrhage. Large haemorrhages may rupture into the cerebral ventricles or out onto the surface of the brain into the subarachnoid space. They occupy space within the brain and cause compression and shift of surrounding brain structures with potentially disastrous effects. Smaller haemorrhages cause less immediate damage and are slowly resorbed. Recovery of function may be surprisingly complete.

The results of surgical treatment of primary intracerebral haemorrhage by drainage of the haematoma are usually disappointing. An important exception arises in cases where the haematoma is in the cerebellum, when surgical intervention may be life-saving.

SUBARACHNOID HAEMORRHAGE

Spontaneous subarachnoid haemorrhage results from the rupture of an intracranial vessel into the subarachnoid space. In the majority of cases the cause is rupture of a berry aneurysm somewhere on or near the circle of Willis. A minority have bled from a congenital arteriovenous malformation.

Clinical features

The clinical features of subarachnoid haemorrhage are often unmistakable. There is a sudden onset of very severe, usually occipital headache which may be accompanied by vomiting, photophobia and a decrease in conscious level. Unless bleeding into the substance of the brain has occurred, focal neurological signs are absent. There are signs of meningism—neck stiffness and a positive Kernig's sign.

Investigation and treatment

Ideally, the first investigation is a CT brain scan. This may demonstrate blood in the subarachnoid space and so confirm the diagnosis. If no CT scanner is available, or the CT scan is negative, a lumbar puncture should be performed. Blood staining of the CSF confirms the diagnosis. Xanthochromia develops within a few hours and persists for two to three weeks.

Management depends on the clinical state of the patient. The aim is to prevent recurrent bleeding by placing a clip on the neck of the aneurysm. If the patient's clinical condition is good, without neurological deficit or persisting reduction in conscious level, many surgeons believe it best to carry out angiography immediately to identify the site of the aneurysm and to procede to early operation. Patients whose condition is poor tolerate angiography badly and surgical morbidity and mortality is high. In such cases investigation is delayed until the patient's condition improves.

SUBDURAL HAEMATOMA

The term subdural haematoma refers to accumulation of blood in the potential space between the arachnoid and the dura. It arises as a result of the rupture of the vessels which carry blood between the superficial veins of the cortex and the venous sinuses running within the dura. The condition may present acutely after head injury when the diagnosis is usually straightforward to establish. A much more difficult diagnostic problem arises in cases where the subdural haematoma has become chronic.

Clinical features

The condition mainly affects infants and the elderly. Patients with ventriculo-atrial or ventriculo-peritoneal CSF shunts are at increased risk. A history of minor head trauma is obtained in about half the cases but the injury is often apparently trivial. Symptoms are non-specific but often include headache, intermittent depression of level of consciousness and confusional states. Signs of a mild hemiparesis may be present.

Investigation

The diagnosis is confirmed by CT brain scan. The radiological signs may be very subtle, especially if haematomas are present bilaterally and no shift of midline structures can be seen.

Treatment

Surgical evacuation of the haematoma through burr holes is required.

16. Epilepsy and loss of consciousness

Epilepsy is defined as recurrent transient attacks of abnormal cerebral function resulting from the excessive discharge of neurones. The clinical manifestations range from a brief disturbance of sensory or motor function to a generalized seizure. About 1 in 50 people suffer an epileptic fit of one sort or another at some time in their lives and in the majority no underlying cause is found. This leads to the idea of a convulsive threshold; all people are potentially at risk of having an epileptic fit but some do so with greater readiness than others. Individuals with a high convulsive threshold have an epileptic fit only under extreme conditions. At the other end of the spectrum, people with a low convulsive threshold may have epileptic fits in the absence of any identifiable provocation.

PATHOGENESIS

The excitability of the neurones of the cerebral cortex is normally held in check by mechanisms of recurrent and collateral inhibition. Following a discharge, a nerve cell inhibits itself and the cells around it from discharging again. The inhibition is short-lived, but long enough to prevent large numbers of neurones discharging synchronously. In epilepsy the mechanisms of inhibition fail to function adequately. A burst of discharges, initially restricted to a few neurones, spreads to surrounding cells giving rise to a state in which large groups of neurones are discharging synchronously and repetitively. If this abnormal activity remains relatively localized, signs and symptoms are restricted to whatever function is associated with that area of cortex and the seizure is partial. Alternatively, the abnormal pattern of neuronal discharge may spread to involve the whole of the cerebral cortex in which case the seizure becomes generalized.

161

A localized area of cortex that is abnormally excitable constitutes an epileptic focus. An epileptic focus is often the result of a structural lesion. The lesion may be benign and non-progressive, for example, an area of cortical gliosis following head injury or birth trauma, or it may be the result of active disease, such as a cerebral tumour or abscess. Epilepsy which is focal in nature should always be regarded as symptomatic of some underlying condition and a patient with focal epilepsy needs to be investigated in order to determine what the cause is.

Many epileptic fits are generalized from the outset and their pathogenesis cannot be explained in terms of a cortical epileptic focus and local failure of inhibitory mechanisms. One view of generalized epilepsy is that the initial event arises in structures deep in the cortex, perhaps the thalamus, and is diffusely projected to the cortex along thalamo-cortical pathways. Recent experimental work in animals, however, suggests that the primary abnormality in generalized epilepsy is a diffuse hyperexcitability of cortical neurones.

In contrast to patients with focal epilepsy, patients with epileptic fits that are generalized from the outset often do not have any identifiable underlying structural lesion. It seems only that their cerebral cortex is unusually excitable and therefore that they have a constitutionally low convulsive threshold.

CLASSIFICATION OF EPILEPSY

The classification of epilepsy set out below (Table 16.1) is adapted from that put forward by the International League against Epilepsy. It is based on the electroencephalographic patterns and clinical features that characterize the attack. The scheme provides a rational framework for thinking about the different types of

Table 16.1 Classification of epilepsy

Generalized (from the onset of the seizure)	Partial
Tonic-clonic (grand mal)	Simple partial seizures (no disturbance of consciousness) Motor Versive
Tonic	Sensory
Akinetic	
Typical absences (petit mal)	Complex partial seizures (consciousness impaired)

Secondary generalization

epilepsy, but it has the defect of failing to take into account the cause of the epilepsy. Another difficulty is that in everyday clinical practice many terms that do not appear in this classification are used by physicians to label the types of seizures of their patients. The solution is to learn the vocabulary of epilepsy in enough detail to understand what is meant whichever terminology is used.

TYPES OF EPILEPTIC SEIZURES

Generalized seizures

Tonic-clonic seizures

These are the commonest form of generalized epileptic seizure and are what the layman usually understands when he hears the term epileptic fit. Tonic clonic seizures are also called *grand mal* fits.

The fit starts with a tonic phase during which all muscle groups are strongly contracted. The tonic contraction can force expiration of air past tense vocal cords and produce an epileptic cry. Consciousness is lost immediately and the patient falls. The arms are held flexed and the legs extended. Teeth are clenched and, because respiratory movements cease, the patient becomes cyanosed. Loss of sphincter control often occurs at this stage. After 10 seconds or so, the tonic phase gives way to the clonic phase. Initially the movements are very rapid in frequency but they gradually slow down to a violent generalized shaking. The tongue may be bitten. The clonic phase lasts from 30 seconds to 2 minutes and then ceases. Deep noisy respirations follow and the patient sleeps.

The effects of a generalized seizure may last several days. Immediately following the fit the patient is confused and sleepy. He may be bruised from his fall and complain of aching muscles. Body temperature is often transiently raised and, if laboratory tests are performed, a leucocytosis and raised plasma concentrations of the muscle enzyme creatinine kinase and the hormone prolactin will be detected.

Tonic seizures

In children seizures consisting of only the tonic phase of the sequence of events described above are quite common. Tonic seizures in adults are very rare.

Akinetic seizures

This is a much less common form of generalized epilepsy in which the patient loses consciousness and falls to the ground, but does not show either tonic or clonic muscle contraction.

Typical absences

Starting in childhood, these attacks consist of a sudden period of blankness sometimes associated with rapid blinking and myoclonic jerks of limbs. Usually the patient does not fall and he is often quite unaware that an attack has occurred. Attacks rarely last more than a few seconds but they may recur frequently. This sort of seizure is also known as *petit mal* epilepsy. A family history of epilepsy is obtained in about half the patients with typical absences.

Typical absence attacks are always accompanied by a characteristic EEG abnormality of regular generalized spike and wave activity at a frequency of 3 Hz. Unless this pattern is present, a diagnosis of typical absence attacks should not be made.

Typical absences only rarely continue beyond adolescence, but in about a third of cases they are replaced by tonic-clonic seizures which persist into adult life.

Partial seizures

Also known as *focal seizures* or *focal fits*, partial seizures are manifestations of epileptic activity that is confined to a localized region of the cerebral cortex. The features of the seizure depend on the area of cortex in which the abnormal activity arises.

Simple motor seizures

Epileptic activity arising in the motor cortex of the frontal lobe causes jerking movements of the contralateral side of the face, limbs or trunk. Occasionally, spread of the epileptic activity through the motor cortex results in a 'march' of the seizure from one muscle group to the next. This is known as Jacksonian epilepsy after Hughlings Jackson who first appreciated its significance. Usually though, the seizure remains confined to one part of the body. Following the seizure, the affected limb may remain weak for several hours—a phenomenon called Todd's paralysis.

If the supplementary motor cortex and centre for voluntary gaze situated in the frontal lobe anterior to the primary motor cortex are involved, the seizure starts with the patient turning his eyes and head away from the side of the lesion. The patient is usually aware of this and can often give a clear account of what happens even if the fit subsequently becomes generalized and consciousness lost. These attacks were once called *adversive seizures* but, because the direction of the forced gaze and deviation of the head is sometimes paradoxical and towards the side of the lesion, they are better labelled *versive* seizures.

Simple sensory seizures

When the epileptic activity arises in the sensory cortex the patient experiences abnormal sensory sensations, often of tingling or numbness, in the contralateral part of the body that corresponds to the region of cortex affected. A sensory march can occur in the same way as for simple motor seizures.

Other simple partial seizures

Simple partial seizures arising in the temporal lobe cause a variety of rather bizarre symptoms. The commonest are olfactory hallucinations, which are usually of an unpleasant odour that the patient may find hard to describe, or a sensation of epigastric discomfort accompanied by a vague but intense feeling that something unpleasant is about to happen. Other symptoms of partial seizures in the temporal lobe include the phenomenon of déjà vu in which the patient feels that he is experiencing something that has happened before, or the inverse—jamais vu—in which he feels that there is something very strange and unfamiliar about his normal surroundings.

Simple partial seizures that involve the occipital lobe are uncommon. They cause primitive visual hallucinations of bright geometric patterns or flashes of light.

Complex partial seizures

Partial seizures that are accompanied by a disturbance of consciousness are known as complex partial seizures to distinguish them from the simple partial seizures described above. The terms *temporal lobe epilepsy* and *psychomotor epilepsy* are also used to refer to this sort of attack. They usually arise in one of the temporal lobes or, less commonly, in a frontal lobe, but EEG recordings during attacks have shown that seizure activity spreads beyond the immediate region of the epileptic focus. Since consciousness is impaired, it would be predicted that the ascending reticular formation at least, becomes involved.

The fit often starts with feelings of altered perception, a disagreeable epigastric sensation or olfactory hallucinations as described for simple partial seizures of the temporal lobe. This phase of the attack is known as the *aura*. As the epileptic activity spreads the patient stares blankly and fails to respond to questions or commands. He may make repeated lip-smacking movements or other facial grimacings. This phase is followed by a short period of semi-purposeful automatic behaviour. Such behaviour usually consists only of hand gestures or apparently aimless perambulation, but occasionally while in this state patients travel considerable distances and have even been known to drive themselves in a car. Postictally the patient is amnesic for the period of the seizure. He often complains of a headache and may be confused and sleepy.

Secondary generalization

The epileptic activity in partial seizures is localized to one region of cerebral cortex at the onset of the fit, but it can spread from the site of origin to involve the whole of the cortex of both hemispheres causing the seizure to become generalized. The process by which localized epileptic activity spreads to involve the whole of the cerebral cortex is known as secondary generalization. The speed with which it occurs varies between individuals and, though usually taking many seconds, secondary generalization may be very abrupt. In such cases, unless an EEG is being recorded at the time, the fact that the initial epileptic activity is localized cannot be observed because the seizure appears generalized from the outset.

CAUSES OF EPILEPSY

Epilepsy is frequently a symptom of some underlying neurological disease and a diagnosis of epilepsy by itself is inadequate. Not only must the type of seizure be established, but the reason why the patient is having seizures must also be understood.

Primary generalized epilepsy

A significant number of patients develop generalized epilepsy in childhood, adolesence or young adult life without any apparent cause. There may be a family history of epilepsy and it is assumed that the underlying reason for their seizures is that they have inherited a low convulsive threshold. By definition, the term primary generalized epilepsy means that no structural reason for the epilepsy is present. Both tonic-clonic seizures and typical absences can be manifestations of primary generalized epilepsy.

Tumours

Seizures which are of focal origin, or which occur for the first time in adult life should always raise the suspicion of a cerebral tumour, particularly if clinical examination reveals abnormal neurological signs.

Cerebrovascular disease

Epilepsy which first starts in late adult life is quite commonly a sequel to cerebral infarction. A less common vascular cause of epilepsy is the presence of an arteriovenous malformation.

Degenerative neurological disease

Fits may occur in a number of degenerative conditions and inborn errors of metabolism:

1. Late stages of Alzheimer's disease
2. Multiple sclerosis
3. Cerebral lipidoses
4. Creutzfeldt-Jakob disease.

Infection and inflammation

Fits are a common feature of infection and inflammation within the central nervous system:

1. Encephalitis
2. Cerebral abscess
3. Subdural empyema
4. Cortical venous thrombosis.

Trauma

Trauma to the head, especially if repeated, or if there has been a depressed skull fracture, a dural tear, or an intracranial haematoma, often results in epilepsy. There may be a latent period of months or even years between the trauma and the first fit.

Drugs

Several drugs lower the convulsive threshold and may cause fits in susceptible individuals:

1. Phenothiazines
2. Tricyclic antidepressants
3. Amphetamines.

Withdrawal from drugs and alcohol

Fits may be precipitated by withdrawal from long-term treatment with benzodiazepines and barbiturates. Abstinence from alcohol in a patient accustomed to a high intake can also cause fits. They are most likely to occur between one and five days after stopping drinking.

Metabolic causes

Metabolic disturbances may be associated with fits:

1. Hypoglycaemia
2. Hyponatraemia
3. Renal failure
4. Hepatic failure.

Pyrexia

High pyrexia in children under the age of 5 years is not uncommonly accompanied by a seizure. In most cases the fits only occur in association with a pyrexial illness and stop spontaneously as the child gets older, but a proportion of cases go on to have afebrile seizures. Prolonged febrile convulsions in children are thought to cause anoxic damage to the temporal lobes and this may be an underlying cause of temporal lobe epilepsy in later life.

STATUS EPILEPTICUS

This term refers to a succession of tonic-clonic seizures without the patient recovering consciousness between seizures. Status epilepticus may complicate any form of epilepsy and it may not always be possible to determine what precipitated it. Sometimes status epilepticus follows a change in drug treatment or withdrawal of anticonvulsants. It may also occur as the presenting feature of a cerebral tumour, cerebral abscess or other intracranial pathology.

Status epilepticus must be considered as a medical emergency. If the fits are allowed to continue there is a serious risk that the patient will become anoxic and pyrexial with resulting permanent brain damage or circulatory collapse. Management of the condition requires several simultaneous lines of attack and, if possible, the patient should be cared for in an intensive care unit.

Initial control of the epilepsy can usually be achieved with an intravenous injection of 10 mg diazepam. The duration of action of this drug is short and as soon as the seizures are controlled, treatment with a longer acting drug such as phenytoin should be started. If this regimen fails to control the fits, paraldehyde may be tried. As a last resort, an infusion of thiopentone can be given, but because of its depressive effects on respiration the patient will need to be ventilated.

General supportive care is of equal importance to attaining control of the epilepsy. The airway must be secured and adequate arterial oxygenation ensured by monitoring of blood gases. Circulatory support with intravenous fluids is required. Most anticonvulsants have a hypotensive effect and frequent checks on blood pressure and pulse rate are essential. Plasma electrolyte and glucose concentrations should be estimated urgently and any metabolic imbalance treated. Pyrexia should be treated with fans and tepid sponging.

Continuous partial epilepsy

This unusual variant of status epilepticus is a result of continuous epileptic activity that remains confined to a localized region of the cortex. In partial motor status, also known as epilepsia partialis continua, there is continuous twitching and jerking of all or part of one side of the body. An underlying structural lesion is invariably present. Treatment with anticonvulsants is usually effective in controlling seizure activity.

Continuous partial epilepsy may also occur in temporal lobe epilepsy. The patient appears confused and unresponsive but because there is no jerking of limbs the diagnosis is far from obvious. Patients with this condition are often initially thought to be drunk or suffering from a drug overdose. Continuous temporal lobe epilepsy is not very common but the diagnosis should always be suspected in a known epileptic presenting with a confusional state. An EEG will confirm the diagnosis.

THE DIFFERENTIAL DIAGNOSIS OF EPILEPSY

Episodes of loss of consciousness are a frequent reason for patients to present at a neurological clinic. Epilepsy is only one of the possible diagnoses to be considered.

Syncope

This term describes a transient episode of loss of consciousness resulting from a brief reduction in cerebral blood perfusion. There is often some precipitating event, such as a prolonged period of standing or an emotional shock. Symptoms of light-headedness, ringing in the ears and nausea usually precede the attack. Witnesses describe the patient as looking pale and then collapsing limply to the ground.

Urinary incontinence may occur in a syncopal attack and if misguided attempts are made by onlookers to keep the patient in an upright posture the cerebral ischaemia may become prolonged enough to cause convulsive movements. If these phenomena occur it may be difficult to decide whether the cause of the episode of loss of consciousness was syncope or epilepsy.

Syncope may also occur in prolonged coughing attacks and, especially in men with a degree of bladder outflow obstruction, with micturition.

Cardiac disease

Disorders of cardiac rhythm which lead to a drop in cardiac output are a common reason for loss of consciousness in the middle aged and elderly. Bradyarrhythmias arising from disease of the cardiac conducting system or from excessive sensitivity of the carotid sinus are more likely to lead to loss of consciousness than tachyarrhythmias. Syncope on exertion is characteristic of aortic stenosis.

Hypoglycaemia

Profound hypoglycaemia will lead to loss of consciousness and occasionally frank epileptic seizures. Symptoms of hypoglycaemia, a feeling of hunger and muscular weakness accompanied by sweating, tachycardia and tremulousness, usually precede loss of consciousness.

Spontaneous hypoglycaemia is rare except in patients who have undergone gastric surgery. These patients may become hypoglycaemic 1−2 hours after a meal because rapid gastric emptying into the jejunum stimulates excessive secretion of insulin.

Insulin-dependent diabetics may, of course, become hypoglycaemic if they miss a meal or take unplanned exercise, but this is rarely a source of diagnostic difficulty.

Tumours which secrete insulin or substances with insulin-like activity, such as insulinomas and retroperitoneal sarcomas, are very rare but often difficult to diagnose.

Hysterical fits

This rather unsatisfactory term refers to attacks of apparent loss of consciousness associated with irregular jerking of the limbs, but rarely with incontinence of urine or tongue biting. The patient's behaviour during a hysterical attack can be influenced by physical restraint or by suggestions from observers. If an attempt is made to test the corneal reflex for example, the patient often screws up his eyes tightly and turns his head away. Hysterical fits occur most commonly in disturbed adolescents. They are also sometimes seen in epileptic patients who are trying to manipulate their relatives or their doctors and the diagnosis may be particularly difficult in these circumstances.

It is not usually helpful to regard such attacks as deliberate malingering but neither, of course, are anticonvulsants of any value in controlling the attacks.

INVESTIGATION OF EPILEPSY

Standard haematological and biochemical tests are usually recommended in all patients with epilepsy to detect any underlying metabolic disorder. Some neurologists also check serology for syphilis. In the absence of any clinical suspicion of abnormality the value of these investigations is small.

An ECG should be performed if there is any indication that attacks of loss of consciousness are of cardiac origin.

An EEG may provide useful information about the type of epilepsy but it is essential to remember that a significant proportion of patients who definitely suffer from epilepsy show no abnormality on an EEG recorded between seizures. A normal EEG does not exclude a diagnosis of epilepsy.

If the epilepsy is focal in nature or focal signs are found on clinical neurological examination, or the EEG shows a focal abnormality, a CT brain scan should be performed to detect any underlying structural lesion.

Cases of epilepsy of late onset, that is after adolescence, should also have a CT brain scan. CT scanning is not usually necessary in children or adolescents who present with generalized epilepsy.

TREATMENT OF EPILEPSY

When and who to treat

Treatment for epilepsy is directed at preventing further seizures. Once started, anticonvulsant medication must be continued for a long period. Because of the long-term implications of starting treatment most neurologists take the view that, while a patient who has had only one fit may well need to be investigated, anticonvulsants should be started only if he has a second fit.

When to stop treatment

A difficult problem arises when an epileptic patient taking anticonvulsants has been free of fits for several years. It is not possible to be sure whether the reason for the absence of fits is because the drug is completely suppressing the tendency to epilepsy, or because he no longer has any need for treatment. The only way to find out is to withdraw the drug and see if his fits recur. Because having a further fit may have serious consequences for a patient's employment, especially if it involves driving a car, he may prefer to continue taking anticonvulsants indefinitely. On the other hand he may so dislike the idea of lifelong medication that he is prepared to take the risk of having another fit to discover if the treatment is still required. Some guidelines can be given: patients whose seizures began in childhood, who have experienced only a few primary generalized seizures and who responded well to the first anticonvulsant, have the best chance of remaining free from fits. Patients with partial seizures and secondary generalization and with persistently abnormal EEGs have a high rate of relapse when anticonvulsants are withdrawn.

Drugs

Drug treatment for epilepsy should be started with a single anticonvulsant. If, after obtaining satisfactory plasma concentrations of the drug, this fails to control the fits another anticonvulsant can be substituted. The first drug should be slowly withdrawn as the second is introduced. Abrupt changes in anticonvulsant medication should be avoided and only in exceptional circumstances should patients take more than one anticonvulsant at a time.

Sodium valproate

This drug is used mainly for the treatment of generalized epilepsy. It is effective in suppressing both typical absences (petit mal) and tonic-clonic seizures. It increases levels of the inhibitory neurotransmitter GABA, but whether its anti-convulsant effects depend on this property is unclear. The plasma half-life is short, but since the drug is lipid soluble plasma levels do not give a clear indication of its concentration in the CNS and the value of monitoring of plasma concentrations as a guide to dosage is limited. Adverse effects include nausea, tremor and hair loss, but these are rare. A few patients taking sodium valproate in combination with other anticonvulsants have developed a fatal hepatic failure.

Carbamazepine

This is the drug of first choice in the treatment of partial seizures. It may also be effective in treating generalized seizures. Treatment should be started at a low dose and increased only gradually to avoid adverse effects of sedation, light-headedness and diplopia. The plasma half-life of the drug is as short as 8 hours in some patients and the drug should be given in divided doses in an attempt to maintain stable plasma concentrations. Even so, large fluctuations may occur and transient diplopia during peaks can be a troublesome side-effect. Monitoring of plasma drug levels is helpful in achieving optimal dosage.

More severe adverse effects of allergic skin reactions and leucopenia require that the drug is withdrawn.

Phenytoin

Phenytoin is effective in tonic-clonic epilepsy and in partial seizures but is not of value in the treatment of typical absences. The therapeutic ratio is small and liver enzymes which metabolize phenytoin become fully saturated at low doses. A small increase in dose can cause a disproportionate increase in plasma concentration of the drug. Monitoring of plasma concentrations is therefore essential to ensure that the drug is being given at the correct dose for the individual patient. The plasma half-life is long and once-daily dosage regimens are satisfactory for most patients. Adverse effects of chronic treatment are hypertrophy of the gums, acne, coarsening of facial features and hirsutism. At toxic levels ataxia, nystagmus, confusion and a paradoxical worsening of epileptic control may occur.

Ethosuximide

The use of this drug is now mainly as a second-line treatment for typical absences.

Barbiturates

Phenobarbitone is an effective anticonvulsant in both generalized and partial epilepsy but it has the adverse effect in many patients of being strongly sedating. It is now rarely instituted as a treatment for epilepsy, but some patients with long-standing epilepsy have had their fits well controlled by it for many years and in such cases it is usually inadvisable to attempt to change to an alternative drug.

Primidone is a related drug that is largely metabolized to phenobarbitone in the body.

Surgery

In very carefully selected patients with intractable epilepsy originating in the temporal lobe, temporal lobectomy can improve seizure control. Patients are more likely to benefit from surgery if an underlying structural abnormality—tumour, arteriovenous malformation, hamartoma—is present.

EPILEPSY AND ACTIVITIES OF DAILY LIFE

Driving

It is a legal requirement that patients with a disability that affects their fitness as a driver inform the Drivers Medical Branch, DVLC, Swansea. This instruction is printed on every driving licence. Patients with epilepsy must be told that they should not drive and they should be reminded of the necessity to inform DVLC, Swansea and their insurance company. Usually, the licence will be restored after two years without fits have passed. If there was a clear precipitating factor and the patient has had a solitary fit and the reason for the fit is not likely to recur the licence may be returned sooner.

No one who has had a fit after the age of three years may ever hold a public services or heavy goods vehicle or aircraft pilot's licence.

Occupation and recreation

Occupations that involve working at heights or with unguarded machinery are clearly unsuitable for patients with epilepsy. The armed forces and the police force will not recruit anyone with a history of seizures in adult life. Apart from these restrictions, the majority of epileptics whose fits are well controlled by anticonvulsant drugs are able to continue in their normal employment. The Employment Advisory Medical Service, a branch of the Health and Safety Executive, is very skilled in persuading employers to adopt a constructive approach to epileptic patients and, with the patient's permission, it is often helpful to refer difficult cases to them.

Patients should be advised against certain pursuits like rock climbing and subaqua diving in which having a fit might be fatal but, with sensible precautions, few sports and leisure-time activities are incompatible with epilepsy.

Pregnancy

The effect of pregnancy on epileptic control is variable. Patients whose epilepsy is poorly controlled before pregnancy often suffer an increase in the frequency of seizures, but in the majority epilepsy is not usually a reason for advising against undertaking a pregnancy.

There is evidence that most of the commonly used anticonvulsants are mildly teratogenic and the incidence of congenital abnormalities is slightly higher in the children of epileptic mothers. Most of these abnormalities are very minor and, because seizures themselves may be harmful to the fetus, the balance of benefit and risk is usually in favour of continuing anticonvulsants. Frequent monitoring of plasma anticonvulsant levels should be carried out because the optimum dose may alter during pregnancy.

Unless both parents are epileptic the chances of the child being affected by epilepsy are very small.

17. Infections of the central nervous system

MENINGITIS

Meningitis is a condition of inflammation of the membranes surrounding the brain and spinal cord—the arachnoid and pia—caused by bacterial, viral or fungal infection, or, much more rarely, by chemical irritation.

Bacterial meningitis

Bacterial meningitis is very much commoner in infants and young children than it is in adults, but at all ages mortality and morbidity are considerable and are often related to delay in diagnosis and treatment. Acute meningitis presents with severe headache, photophobia and high pyrexia. The patient feels extremely unwell and may be drowsy and confused. There are signs of meningeal irritation: neck stiffness, neck retraction and a positive Kernig's sign (see Fig. 9.1). If there has been delay in seeking medical attention the patient may be unconscious but this is not an early feature. Focal neurological signs do not occur in meningitis unless the infection has spread into the substance of the brain—meningoencephalitis—or the meningitis is secondary to a brain abscess.

The usual clinical features of acute bacterial meningitis are often obscured if the patient has been recently treated with oral antibiotics. These may modify the infection but fail to eradicate it and, unless the signs of meningeal irritation are carefully looked for, the diagnosis will be missed.

Viral meningitis

Viral meningitis is usually a much milder illness than bacterial meningitis. The speed of onset is slower with a prodromal phase of a pyrexial illness that may be associated with a rash and sore throat.

Common organisms causing acute meningitis

Bacteria

The three commonest bacteria causing meningitis are:

1. *Haemophilus influenzae*
2. *Neisseria meningitidis*
3. *Streptococcus pneumoniae.*

H. influenzae predominates in children while *Neisseria meningitidis* and *Streptococcus pneumoniae* are more frequent in adults. In neonates *E. coli* is not uncommonly the causal organism.

A large number of other organisms are occasionally responsible, including *Streptococcus pyogenes* and *Staphylococcus aureus*. Infection with *Leptospira* species sometimes produces a predominantly meningitic illness. *Listeria monocytogenes* should be considered, especially if the patient is immunosuppressed. Patients who have had a CSF shunt inserted are liable to infection with *Staphylococcus albus*.

Viruses

Echovirus is the commonest cause of aseptic meningitis. Other viruses which may be responsible are mumps virus and Coxsackie viruses.

Diagnosis

Confirmation of a clinical diagnosis of meningitis requires urgent bacteriological and biochemical analysis of the CSF. Unless the patient is unconscious or focal neurological signs are present, a lumbar puncture must be performed and the specimens taken to the laboratory for immediate analysis. If the patient is unconsciousness or shows focal neurological signs a CT brain scan is needed to exclude the presence of an obstructive hydrocephalus which would render a lumbar puncture dangerous. It is crucial that no unnecessary delay results from having to organize this investigation.

Typical CSF findings in bacterial meningitis are summarized in Table 17.1.

Table 17.1   Typical CSF values in bacterial meningitis

Apperance	Cloudy or frankly purulent
Pressure	Raised
Cell count	Raised, 100–10 000 polymorphs
Glucose	< 2.5 mmol/l (often undetectable)
Protein	> 0.8 mg/l
Gram stain	Organisms seen and identified

The initial bacteriological diagnosis can usually be made from a Gram-stained CSF film and is subsequently confirmed by culture of CSF. Blood cultures are positive in about half the cases of acute bacterial meningitis.

Viral meningitis is characterized by an increased cell count (50–1000 cells per ml) of lymphocytes or monocytes. Protein concentrations may be raised but glucose concentrations are normal.

Treatment

If a bacterial cause for the meningitis is suspected, treatment with parenteral antibiotics must be started as soon as possible. Delay in identification of the responsible organism should never be allowed to delay treatment. If the organism is not known, intravenous treatment with both benzyl penicillin and chloramphenicol is recommended. Antibiotics should not be given intrathecally.

Following positive identification of the organism, specific antibiotic treatment should be discussed with a bacteriologist. Usual recommendations for the commoner organisms causing meningitis are given in Table 17.2.

Intravenous fluids will be necessary to maintain adequate hydration. Some degree of inappropriate secretion of ADH often ac-

Table 17.2   Recommended antibiotic treatment for bacterial meningitis in adults

Organism	Antibiotic
Neisseria meningitidis	Benzyl penicillin 2 grams 2-hourly i.v.
Haemophilus influenzae	Chloramphenicol 1.2 grams 6-hourly i.v.
Streptococcus pneumoniae	Benzyl penicillin 2 grams 2-hourly i.v.

These recommendations apply only to adults. In children, dosage must be modified according to age and weight.

companies meningitis and plasma electrolytes must be carefully monitored.

Viral meningitis is usually a benign and self-limiting condition. Treatment is symptomatic.

Chronic meningitis

Infection of the meninges with tubercle bacillus, syphilis or the fungus *Cryptococcus neoformans* and chronic meningeal inflammation from granulomatous or vasculitic disease produces a clinical picture that differs from that of acute meningitis. In these conditions the meninges around the brain stem and the base of the brain tend to be most severely affected. This may result in obstruction to the normal flow of CSF and cause hydrocephalus, damage cranial nerves running along the base of the brain or provoke endarteritis causing infarction of brain stem and spinal cord.

The clinical features are non-specific and insidious in their onset. Fever and meningism are usually present and in addition there may be seizures, papilloedema, focal neurological signs and cranial nerve palsies.

Tuberculous meningitis

Attempts to confirm the diagnosis are made by examining the CSF. Typically, the protein concentration is considerably elevated at $1-4$ g/l and the glucose concentration reduced below 50% of blood glucose concentration. Acid-fast bacilli are often not seen on microscopy and are only revealed after prolonged culture. In a significant proportion of cases no organisms are ever isolated, but even in these a trial of antituberculous chemotherapy may be worthwhile.

Treatment. Treatment should not await isolation of the organism. Choice of antituberculous chemotherapy requires expert advice but is likely to include streptomycin, isoniazid and ethambutol. Steroids are often given in the hope that endarteritis and basal arachnoiditis will be minimized.

Other causes of chronic meningitis

Fungal meningitis occurs as an opportunistic infection in immunosuppressed patients. In the UK the commonest organism is *Cryptococcus neoformans*. Diagnosis is often extremely difficult, but the organism may be identified if the CSF is stained with Indian ink. Treatment is given with antifungal agents such as amphotericin B.

The diagnosis of syphilitic meningitis is made serologically. Treatment is with benzyl penicillin.

Granulomatous meningitis as a result of sarcoidosis is treated with steroids.

Parameningeal infection

Subdural empyema

This is a rare but very serious complication of infection of the paranasal sinuses. In the majority of cases the frontal sinuses are the site of primary infection, though often the infection is subclinical. The infection spreads intracranially through the thin bony wall of the sinus and a layer of pus forms over one frontal lobe. The organisms responsible are often anaerobes or microaerophilic bacteria (*Streptococcus milleri*), but may be *Staphylococcus aureus* or *E. coli*.

Clinical signs. The patient is extremely unwell with a high fever and a severe frontal or generalized headache. Focal features, such as cranial nerve palsies, hemiplegia and, if the dominant hemisphere is affected, dysphasia, are frequent and seizures may occur. Meningism is almost invariable and papilloedema is common. The diagnosis can usually be confirmed by CT scan but, because the collection of pus may be of the same X-ray density as normal brain, interpretation may be difficult. Urgent neurosurgical intervention is required to drain the pus and this must be followed by parenteral treatment with antibiotics.

Venous sinus and cortical vein thrombosis

Pyogenic infection of the middle ear and mastoid air cells may result in osteitis of the surrounding bone and secondary thrombosis of the lateral sinus. The veins of the face and orbit communicate with the intracranial venous drainage and infections of the face may be complicated by infective thrombosis of the cavernous sinus. Thrombosis of cortical veins may occur as a complication of bacterial meningitis or as a result of a generalized coagulopathy. All these conditions are rare. Treatment is directed at the underlying infection. Whether the benefits of anticoagulation in this situation outweigh the dangers is unknown.

Spinal epidural abscess

Epidural abscess is a rare metastatic complication of pyogenic infection elsewhere in the body. The patient presents with fever, severe back pain and signs of spinal cord compression. Myelography is necessary to confirm the diagnosis and treatment by surgical decompression and antibiotics should be prompt.

Intracerebral abscess

Direct spread of infection from middle ear and paranasal sinuses, or blood-borne spread from chronic lung infection or bacterial endocarditis occasionally gives rise to abscess formation within the substance of the brain. The commonest site is in the subcortical white matter. The abscess develops gradually and a period of cerebritis precedes the formation of a mature abscess. Anaerobic organisms and *Streptococcus viridans* are the common culprits.

Clinical signs

The insidious onset of symptoms and signs makes the diagnosis difficult. Pyrexia, which may be intermittent, evidence of raised intracranial pressure, focal neurological signs whose nature depends on the site of the abscess and epilepsy are the commonest features. Signs of sinus or ear infection, a history of recent head injury, or evidence of lung infection or endocarditis in a patient who develops neurological signs should always raise the possibility of a cerebral abscess.

Treatment

The diagnosis is confirmed by a CT brain scan. Treatment consists of antibiotics which should include metronidazole and benzyl penicillin, and surgical drainage. A careful search for the source of infection and treatment to eradicate it is also required. Prognosis depends heavily on early diagnosis and treatment. Even with prompt treatment mortality is as high as 10% and many survivors have persisting focal deficits.

Encephalitis, encephalomyelitis and myelitis

Acute viral encephalitis

In the UK the most important cause of acute viral encephalitis is

Herpes simplex type 1. This organism produces a severe necrotizing encephalitis which affects particularly the temporal and frontal lobes. Symptoms of headache and fever progress, over a few days, to impairment of consciousness and seizures. Focal signs may be present. Unless brain biopsy is undertaken, isolation of the virus is not usually achieved and serological studies can only be interpreted in retrospect. The EEG shows high-amplitude slow-wave activity and a CT scan may demonstrate low density areas in the frontal and temporal lobes.

Untreated, the condition has a high mortality. The antiviral agent acyclovir, which inhibits viral DNA synthesis, is currently the best treatment but a large proportion of the survivors are left with severe memory impairment and other intellectual deficits.

Mumps virus can also cause an acute encephalitic illness, but the prognosis for recovery is usually good. Several other viruses including influenza virus, Epstein-Barr virus, Coxsackie virus and, in the United States and South America, togaviruses may cause encephalitis on rare occasions.

Postinfectious encephalitis

Also known as acute disseminated encephalomyelitis, this is a rare sequel to a number of exanthematous viral infections including measles, rubella and chickenpox. Estimates of the frequency of this complication vary, but it seems to be less frequent than 1 in 1000 cases of primary infection. One to three weeks after the onset of the infectious illness there is an abrupt onset of a pyrexial illness associated with a decrease in conscious level, headache, pyramidal, cerebellar and brain stem signs and sometimes convulsions. The mechanism seems to involve a hypersensitivity reaction rather than viral invasion of the central nervous system and pathologically there are numerous foci of demyelination in a perivascular distribution. Mortality is over 20% and many of the cases who survive are left with neurological deficits. Treatment with steroids in high doses may be of benefit.

Subacute sclerosing panencephalitis (SSPE)

Another very uncommon complication of measles infection is SSPE. The condition is a result of persistence of virus in the brain following an attack of measles. There is a slow progression of the disease over 2–18 months characterized by intellectual deterioration, myoclonus and epilepsy. The disease is usually fatal.

Paralytic poliomyelitis

Although this is now an extremely rare disease in the Western world it remains common in developing countries. Polio virus is an enterovirus spread by the faecal−oral route. In the majority of cases the infection is subclinical with the virus localized to the tonsils and the lymphoid tissue of the gut. In a minority, a viraemic phase follows about 10 days after the initial infection. Non-specific symptoms of fever and malaise occur. The infection may abort at this stage or spread to the central nervous system.

Even when the virus involves the central nervous system, the majority of cases develop a non-paralytic meningitic illness characterized by fever, malaise and meningism. Only a very small proportion, of the order of 0.01%–0.1% of non-immune people exposed to the virus, develop paralytic poliomyelitis. The paralytic form of the disease starts with fever and aching pains in the muscles. Weakness, which is often assymetrical, develops over a few days. Limb muscles are most frequently involved but bulbar and respiratory musculature may also be affected. Once the progression of the weakness has stopped, recovery starts. The degree of recovery is variable and improvement may continue for many months.

The virus preferentially attacks the anterior horn cells in the spinal cord and this accounts for the lower motor neurone signs that dominate the clinical picture.

Progressive multifocal leucoencephalopathy

Chronically immunosuppressed patients, particularly cases of reticuloses or AIDS, are vulnerable to infection of the central nervous system with Papovavirus. The virus invades oligodendroglial cells and causes demyelination of white matter. The clinical features are of a progressive neurological deterioration over a few months with hemiparesis, cortical blindness, dementia and epilepsy. A few cases have been reported to respond to cytarabine, but in most cases the disease ends in death.

AIDS

Infection with human immunodeficiency virus (HIV) can cause a whole range of neurological disturbances from cognitive impairment, memory loss and acute psychotic states to cerebellar and corticospinal tract degeneration. Some of these effects are a direct result of the presence of the virus in the brain and some are a consequence of opportunistic infection of the central nervous system secondary to HIV-mediated immunodeficiency.

HIV involves the central nervous system at an early stage of the infection but there may be a long latent period before the effects of the virus are manifested. Patients who are HIV positive and who show signs of neurological disease should be fully investigated in order to exclude any treatable secondary infection. Cryptococcal meningitis, progressive multifocal leucoencephalopathy and herpes simplex encephalitis are some of the commoner causes of secondary infection.

The immunosuppressive effects of HIV infection also predispose to the development of lymphomas of the central nervous system.

HERPES ZOSTER

First exposure to the herpes zoster virus results in chickenpox. Except in the rare cases of fulminating infection in immunosuppressed patients, full recovery from chickenpox is almost invariable. However, the virus is not eliminated; it persists in the dorsal root ganglia and, many years later often for no apparent reason, there may be a recrudescence of the infection localized to the distribution of one or two nerve roots—an attack of *shingles*.

Severe pain in a dermatomal distribution precedes the development of a vesicular rash by a day or two. The appearance of the vesicles is identical to that of chickenpox except that they are restricted to a dermatomal distribution. The rash subsides after 10 days. In older patients, pain in the distribution of the former rash may continue indefinitely—a condition known as post-herpetic neuralgia.

18. Intracranial neoplasms

Primary neoplasms of the central nervous system, which may arise from any of the cell types represented there, account for about 10% of all primary neoplasms in man. In adults the commonest primary intracranial tumours are astrocytomas and meningiomas, the majority of which are supratentorial. In children the pattern is reversed; most tumours are infratentorial and are either cerebellar astrocytomas or medulloblastomas. Distant metastases from intracranial tumours are exceptionally rare and, by a definition of malignancy which includes a propensity to metastasize, most of these neoplasms are benign. However, because the skull forms a rigid and more or less inexpansible compartment, any lesion inside it can grow only by compressing and distorting other structures. The consequences of any intracranial space-occupying lesion are potentially malignant no matter how benign its histological appearance.

The brain is a common site for metastatic deposits from other primary tumours and about 20% of all adult intracranial neoplasms are secondary. Almost any primary neoplasm can metastasize to the brain, but those that do so most frequently are carcinomas of lung, breast, stomach, thyroid and kidney.

PATHOLOGY

The World Health Organization classification of tumours shown in Table 18.1 is based on the cell type of origin of the tumour. Many of the types of tumour are extremely rare and will be dealt with only briefly.

Astrocytoma

This is the commonest primary brain tumour of adults. The de-

187

Table 18.1   WHO Classification of intracranial neoplasms

Cell type of origin	Tumour
Neuroepithelial	Astrocytoma
	Oligodendroglioma
	Ependymoma
	Choroid plexus papilloma
	Pineocytoma and pineoblastoma
	Tumours of neural origin:
	ganglioglioma
	gangliocytoma
	neuroblastoma
	Tumours of embryonic origin: medulloblastoma
Meningeal	Meningioma
	Meningeal sarcoma
Nerve sheath	Neurilemmoma
	Neurofibroma
Blood vessels	Haemangioblastoma
Germ cells	Germinoma
	Teratoma
Maldevelopment	Craniopharyngioma
	Dermoid and epidermoid cyst
	Colloid cyst
Anterior pituitary	Adenoma
	Carcinoma
Miscellaneous	Chordoma
	Chemodectoma
	Primary malignant lymphoma
Metastatic	Lung
	Kidney
	Thyroid, etc.

gree of malignancy, based on histological criteria of mitotic rate, degree of differentiation, cellularity and vascular proliferation, varies and they are subdivided into four grades. Grades 3 and 4, the most malignant, are unfortunately the most frequently encountered. Ninety per cent of astrocytomas arise in the frontal, parietal or occipital lobes and the remaining 10% in the corpus callosum, thalamus, occipital lobe and brain stem.

Oligodendroglioma

Much less common than astrocytomas, these tumours are usually slow growing and relatively benign. They have a tendency to calcify and this feature may be visible on a plain skull X-ray.

Medulloblastoma

This is a rapidly growing glioma which usually occurs as a midline cerebellar tumour in children.

Ependymoma

These tumours arise from the ependymal cells lining the ventricles and central canal of the spinal cord. The majority occur in the fourth ventricle.

Meningioma

Meningiomas are benign tumours arising, as the name indicates, from the membranes surrounding the brain. They are commoner in women than in men and are unusual before late middle age. Most frequently they arise over the convexity of the hemispheres or parasagittally from the falx. They can also occur in the basal regions, in the olfactory groove of the anterior fossa, on the greater wing of the sphenoid and around the pituitary fossa.

Pineal tumours

Several tumour types occur in the pineal: pineocytomas, pineoblastomas, teratomas and germinomas. Because of their position, they tend to compress the dorsal part of the midbrain in the region of the superior colliculi. This causes failure of conjugate upward gaze and loss of the pupillary light reflex, a pair of signs which goes under the eponym of Parinaud's syndrome. These tumours frequently interrupt and block the outward flow of CSF from the ventricular system and cause hydrocephalus.

Pituitary tumours

Adenomas of the anterior lobe of the pituitary form about 5% of all intracranial tumours. Frequently, they are secretory and present with endocrine symptoms and signs. As they enlarge they expand the pituitary fossa and by extending upwards compress the optic chiasm. This results in a characteristic visual field defect—a bitemporal hemianopia.

The anterior part of the pituitary develops from the primitive mouth cavity. Embryonic cell rests left behind during development have the potential to become neoplastic giving rise to a craniopharyngioma—a cystic tumour without endocrine function itself, but able to impair normal hypothalamic regulation of pituitary secretions.

Chordomas

These are rare tumours which arise from primitive notochord remnants. Most occur in the sacrococcygeal region but some are found arising from the clivus, the posterior part of the sphenoid bone.

CLINICAL FEATURES

Raised intracranial pressure

Because of their space-occupying effect and their ability to interfere with the flow and resorption of CSF raised intracranial pressure frequently accompanies intracranial neoplasms. The following signs and symptoms suggest raised intracranial pressure.

Headache

A poorly localized headache, sometimes quite severe, which tends to be worst on waking and exacerbated by bending, stooping and straining is probably the result of stretching of the dura and intracranial blood vessels.

Papilloedema

Swelling of the optic disc, is a common but not invariable accompaniment of raised intracranial pressure. It is thought that the raised pressure in the subarachnoid space which surrounds the optic nerve interferes with venous and lymphatic drainage from the retina and the nerve itself. An additional factor may be impairment of axoplasmic flow in the fibres of the optic nerve. Transient obscuration of vision may occur when papilloedema is present, especially with manoeuvres which raise ICP still further, like bending or straining. Rarely, prolonged papilloedema results in permanent visual loss.

Vomiting

Sudden vomiting, often without a preceding feeling of nausea, may occur soon after waking when the headache is at its worst. This symptom is probably caused by compression of vomiting centres in the medulla.

Epilepsy

Seizures are common in patients with intracranial neoplasms, particularly if the tumour involves the cerebral cortex. However, the converse is not true; only a minority of patients presenting with late onset epilepsy, probably about 10%, will turn out to harbour a tumour. The chances of a tumour being present are increased if the fits are focal or if the patient presents in status epilepticus. Focal fits may help localize the site of the tumour. For example, a focal motor seizure suggests that the contralateral frontal lobe is involved.

Focal signs and symptoms

As intracranial tumours increase in size they compress and distort surrounding brain tissue and interfere with normal function. Even with rapidly growing tumours, this loss of function is a gradual process and the symptoms which result are usually progressive rather than of sudden onset. Signs and symptoms depend on the site of the tumour and can be predicted from knowledge of localization of function within the central nervous system.

Frontal lobe:

1. Change in personality
2. Intellectual deterioration
3. Contralateral hemiparesis (if motor cortex is involved)
4. Expressive dysphasia (if in the dominant hemisphere)

Parietal lobe:

1. Contralateral sensory loss of cortical type

2. Sensory and visual inattention
3. Receptive dysphasia (if in dominant hemisphere)
4. Apraxia

Temporal lobe

1. Epilepsy
2. Deterioration of memory

Occipital lobe

Contralateral homonymous hemianopia. Supratentorial tumours may enlarge to such an extent that normal brain is displaced from its usual anatomical position. The medial parts of the temporal lobes may be forced downwards through the defect in the tentorium occupied by the mid-brain into the posterior fossa. When this happens the III and VI cranial nerves are stretched over the sharp edge of the tentorium. A palsy of either of these nerves can be an early feature of tentorial herniation.

Cerebellopontine angle tumours

The majority of tumours arising in the cerebellopontine angle are neurilemmomas of the auditory nerve, often known simply as acoustic nerve tumours. The earliest symptoms of deafness and tinnitus are related to damage to the auditory nerve itself. As the tumour enlarges it impinges on the trigeminal nerve causing loss of the corneal reflex and numbness over the face. The facial nerve also lies adjacent but, for some reason, facial palsy is very uncommon. Expansion of the tumour in a medial direction compresses the brain stem and cerebellum giving symptoms of ataxia.

Other rarer causes of tumours in the cerebellopontine angle include neurilemmomas of the trigeminal nerve and meningiomas.

Posterior fossa tumours

Tumours of the posterior fossa tend to obstruct the normal outflow of CSF from the fourth ventricle at an early stage and present with symptoms of raised intracranial pressure or cerebellar signs of ataxia, dysarthria and nystagmus.

INVESTIGATIONS
Skull X-ray

Signs of an intracranial tumour on a plain skull X-ray, if present at all, are usually rather subtle. Calcification in oligodendrogliomas, craniopharyngiomas and meningiomas may be visible. Widening of the internal auditory meatus is a classic sign of an acoustic neuroma. Raised intracranial pressure may show itself as thinning of the dorsum sellae. But most patients with an intracranial tumour have a normal skull X-ray and, as an investigation in cases of suspected tumour, it is far too unreliable to be of much value.

CT scanning

CT scanning with contrast enhancement is highly sensitive in the detection of intracranial tumours and is an essential investigation if such a lesion is suspected. The size of the tumour, its position and its relation to other structures can be delineated and it is often possible to make an accurate prediction about the tumour type.

Angiography

This procedure carries a significant morbidity and mortality and its use is mainly restricted to cases where neurosurgical intervention is contemplated and information about the vascular supply of the tumour is needed to plan the surgical approach.

Biopsy

Biopsy of the tumour, either through a burr-hole or at craniotomy, allows confirmation of the diagnosis and, usually, accurate identification of tumour type. The value of the procedure is debated; although it may prevent a potentially treatable benign tumour being misdiagnosed as a malignant glioma, it carries a very significant morbidity even when carried out by experienced neurosurgeons.

TREATMENT
Surgery

Complete surgical removal of benign tumours can sometimes be achieved, but often only incomplete excision is possible because of the proximity of the tumour to vital brain structures. Meningiomas and acoustic nerve tumours carry the best prognosis.

Malignant gliomas cannot be completely resected because of the infiltrative nature of the tumour. The most that can be hoped for is successful temporary palliation by incomplete removal or internal   decompression.

Radiotherapy

Radiotherapy has been shown to increase the median survival time in malignant gliomas by a few months. The treatment is usually well tolerated but the benefit is often disappointingly small.

Chemotherapy

Some clinical trials have shown a small increase in survival time when patients with malignant gliomas have been treated with CCNU and other cytotoxic agents in combination with surgery and radiotherapy. This benefit is sometimes at the expense of side-effects of prolonged vomiting and marrow suppression. Targeting of tumour tissue using cytotoxic agents bound to monoclonal antibodies with affinity for the tumour offers hope for the future.

Symptomatic

The oedema associated with some malignant gliomas responds to treatment with dexamethasone and symptoms caused by the mass effect of the tumour may be dramatically, though temporarily, improved. Epilepsy complicating cerebral tumour should be treated with anticonvulsants. The insertion of a shunt into the ventricular system is sometimes indicated for the relief of hydrocephalus.

19. Parkinsonism and diseases of the basal ganglia

PARKINSON'S DISEASE

Parkinson's disease was first described by a London general practitioner, James Parkinson, in 1817 in an essay entitled 'The shaking palsy'. It affects people of all races and though it was believed for a long time that the disease was less frequent in negroes, a recent carefully designed epidemiological survey has shown this idea to be false.

Pathology

The main pathological feature is a profound cell loss in a specific population of neurones in the substantia nigra. These cells send a dopaminergic projection to the striatum and consequently, in Parkinson's disease, the dopamine content of the striatum is severely reduced. Abnormalities of dopaminergic transmission and dopamine binding have been discovered in other parts of the brain and deficits of other transmitter systems are also known to exist but these seem to be of secondary importance to the defect in the nigrostriatal pathway. The histological hallmark of Parkinson's disease is the Lewy body—an intracellular inclusion found mainly in the surviving neurones of the substantia nigra.

A syndrome indistinguishable from idiopathic Parkinson's disease, except for the absence of Lewy bodies, has recently been identified in drug addicts who injected themselves with a synthetic opiate contaminated with methylphenyltetrahydropyridine (MPTP). A metabolite of MPTP is specifically neurotoxic to the dopaminergic neurones of the substantia nigra and this discovery has stimulated research into many aspects of the disease. But the overwhelming majority of patients with Parkinson's disease, of course, have never been intravenous drug abusers and the underlying cause of the idiopathic form of the disease remains a mystery.

195

Clinical features

The age of onset is rarely less than 50 years and the incidence of the disease increases with age. The main clinical features are tremor, rigidity, bradykinesia and disturbance of posture.

Tremor

A coarse tremor is present in about 70% of patients. The tremor is present at rest and is sometimes diminished by active movement. It is often asymmetrical in the early stages and almost always affects the hands and arms to a greater extent than the legs. In the hand the tremor characteristically consists of a rhythmic alternating flexion and extension of the fingers and thumb coupled with a rotatory oscillation at the wrist—the pill-rolling tremor. As the disease progresses tremor may spread to involve all limbs and even the muscles of mastication and the tongue. Like most involuntary movements the tremor of Parkinson's disease is made worse by anxiety and emotional stress. It disappears when the patient is asleep.

Rigidity

An increase of muscle tone, more marked in upper than lower limbs, is present. All muscle groups are affected and, unlike the spasticity found in lesions of the corticospinal tract, the increased muscle tone is apparent throughout the whole range of movement of a joint. The degree of rigidity is frequently greater on one side of the body than the other and can be accentuated by asking the patient to perform some voluntary movement with the limb opposite to the one being tested. To an examiner, the sensation of moving the limb of a patient with Parkinson's disease is like bending a lead pipe or, more commonly, since tremor is often superimposed on the rigidity, like moving a lever along a rachet. The term cog-wheel rigidity is used to describe this physical sign.

Bradykinesia

The most disabling feature of Parkinson's disease is bradykinesia—difficulty with the initiation of movement. In its mildest form it may be apparent only as the loss of arm swinging when walking or in the infrequent use of gesture when speaking. When more severe all movements are affected. The patient walks with short shuffling steps, has difficulty maintaining his balance when he turns and always seems to be on the verge of toppling over. His face is expressionless and his speech is both dysarthric and dysphonic. Fine movements of hands and fingers are also affected. The handwriting of a patient with Parkinson's disease is typically very small and shaky.

Disturbance of postural tone and postural reflexes

Patients with Parkinson's disease adopt a stooped posture and hold their limbs in flexion as a result of disturbance of the mechanisms that maintain normal muscle tone. Flexion of the neck is a prominent feature and may be present to such a degree that even when the patient is lying in bed his head is held above the pillow rather than resting on it. The ability to make rapid postural adjustments is lost so that the patient is unable to make rapid changes of direction when moving about and is often in danger of falling.

Other features

The features described above make it very easy to recognize advanced cases of the disease. In the very early stages, however, diagnosis is much more difficult. The presenting symptoms are often very non-specific. The patient may complain of rather vague aches and pains in the muscles of the limbs, especially in the shoulder and upper arm, general fatigue, loss of energy and drive and of feelings of depression. The physical signs at this stage tend to be rather subtle: loss of arm swinging when walking, lack of emotional expression in the face, infrequent blinking and slight cog-wheel rigidity at the wrist, accentuated when the patient is making voluntary movements with the other arm.

In the later stages of the disease disturbance of autonomic function is common. This most often shows itself as postural hypotension and, in male patients, as impotence. There is increasing evidence too, that a significant number of patients suffer intellectual deterioration as the disease progresses.

Treatment

L-dopa

Oral medication with the immediate precursor of dopamine, L-dopa, in combination with benserazide or carbidopa, which prevent the peripheral metabolism of L-dopa, is the mainstay of treatment.

This drug increases the concentration of dopamine in the striatum and has a major effect on the most disabling feature of the disease—bradykinesia—in a very high percentage of patients. Quite why it should work is mysterious; after all, the dopaminergic nerve terminals have largely degenerated and those which remain are presumably not prevented from working by lack of substrate. It may be that the conversion of L-dopa to dopamine takes place in the walls of blood vessels or in glial cells.

Unfortunately, treatment with L-dopa has no effect on the progression of the underlying disease and the efficacy of this drug gradually declines with time. The patient may experience large fluctuations in mobility related to the changing concentrations of striatal dopamine following an oral dose of L-dopa. From being frozen by bradykinesia he may, over the space of a few minutes, become disabled by involuntary dyskinetic movements.

Dopamine agonists

Dopamine agonists, principally bromocriptine, may be useful if the dose-related fluctuations in response to L-dopa cannot be overcome by increasing the frequency of medication with the latter drug.

Anticholinergics

Anticholinergic drugs such as benzhexol and orphenadrine produce a modest reduction in muscular rigidity. They may be used in combination with L-dopa.

Neither anticholinergics nor L-dopa usually have very much effect on tremor. Indeed, L-dopa may sometimes make it worse.

Surgery

Stereotaxic procedures in which small lesions are made in the thalamus or globus pallidus are occasionally performed to treat patients with severe and disabling tremor.

OTHER CAUSES OF A PARKINSONIAN SYNDROME

Drug-induced parkinsonism

Dopamine antagonists such as phenothiazines and haloperidol

may cause a clinical syndrome very like idiopathic Parkinson's disease. This adverse effect is dose related and usually occurs within the first few weeks of treatment. Recovery after withdrawal of the drug may take many months. To avoid misdiagnosing this condition as idiopathic Parkinson's disease all patients presenting with a parkinsonian syndrome should be carefully questioned about their regular medication.

Postencephalitic parkinsonism

In the 1920s there was a widespread epidemic of an encephalitic illness presumed to be viral despite the fact that no causal organism was ever isolated. A parkinsonian syndrome was a frequent sequel to the encephalitis although the onset of symptoms could be delayed for many years after the original illness. A particular feature of postencephalitic parkinsonism is the oculogyric crisis; this is a spasm of conjugate external ocular muscles causing a forced deviation of gaze usually in an upward direction. Very few patients with postencephalitic parkinsonism still survive, but if you encounter one do not miss the opportunity to hear their story.

Other rare causes of a parkinsonian syndrome include *multisystem atrophy*, also known as the Shy-Drager syndrome, in which severe autonomic failure is a major feature, and *progressive supranuclear palsy*, the Steele-Richardson-Olszewski syndrome, in which parkinsonism is accompanied by defects of vertical gaze, progressive dementia and a disturbance of posture leading to hyperextension of the axial skeleton, particularly of the neck. Parkinsonian features may also be found in states of diffuse brain injury such as occur with widespread arteriosclerotic disease and following repeated trauma to the head.

HUNTINGTON'S DISEASE

This is a genetically determined condition, inherited as an autosomal dominant trait, which usually first presents between the ages of 30 and 50. The delayed onset of symptoms means that most patients have completed their families by the time the disease is apparent; their children therefore have to live with the knowledge that there is a 50% chance that they too will subsequently develop the disease. The main clinical features are a progressive dementia associated with involuntary choreiform movements. The disease is characterized pathologically by a decrease in GABA concentrations in the caudate nucleus and putamen and by loss of neurones from the frontal lobes of the cerebral cortex and from the basal ganglia. No form of treatment is known that affects the course of the disease and most patients die within 10–15 years of the onset of symptoms. Genetic counselling to other members of the patient's family is the most constructive approach that can be taken to limit the prevalence of the disease.

WILSON'S DISEASE

This is a rare autosomally recessively inherited abnormality of copper metabolism that prevents the normal excretion of copper in the bile. Affected individuals accumulate the metal in many body tissues but the toxic effect is confined to the brain and the liver. About 50% of cases present with neurological symptoms in late childhood or young adult life. Most of the remainder present in childhood with liver disease. In a few cases the predominant symptoms are psychiatric.

Neurological presentations are characterized by disorders of movement. This may be a syndrome of rigidity and bradykinesia resembling parkinsonism, or the development of involuntary movements with sustained dystonic postures, or tremor. The major pathological features are found in the basal ganglia, especially the putamen and the globus pallidus, where there is cell death, gliosis and cavitation, and in the liver which is cirrhotic.

Investigations

Although very rare, a diagnosis of Wilson's disease should be considered in any young person presenting with an extrapyramidal syndrome (or with hepatic cirrhosis) because effective treatment is available. Measurement of caeruloplasmin, a circulating protein with a high affinity for copper, serum copper levels and urinary copper excretion is usually adequate to confirm or exclude the diagnosis. In Wilson's disease caeruloplasmin concentrations are low, serum copper is reduced and urinary copper excretion is raised. If doubt about the diagnosis remains, liver biopsy for histology and measurement of copper content is necessary. In untreated cases a deposit of copper may be visible on the posterior surface of the cornea at the junction between the cornea and the sclera as a golden brown coloured ring—the Kayser-Fleischer ring. This famous sign can often be seen only by slit-lamp examination.

Treatment

Treatment with the chelating agent D-penicillamine promotes the urinary excretion of copper and, providing the diagnosis has not been too long delayed, will lead to clinical improvement. Untreated, the condition is invariably progressive. Careful monitoring is required partly to ensure that adequate excretion of copper is being achieved and partly because of the possibility of toxic reaction to the drug.

Diagnosis of a case of Wilson's disease should lead to careful screening of the patient's family. Treatment of asymptomatic individuals will prevent the appearance of both neurological and hepatic complications.

DYSTONIA

The dystonias are a group of rare disorders whose clinical manifestations are dominated by sustained muscle contraction. This frequently causes repetitive twisting movements of limbs, trunk or head, or the forced adoption of an abnormal posture. The aetiology and pathology are poorly understood but these conditions are thought to be extrapyramidal in origin.

A generalized dystonia—dystonia musculorum deformans—with onset in childhood or young adult life is characterized by bizarre posturing of head, trunk and limbs. Most cases are sporadic but some may be the result of a genetic defect.

The commonest partial dystonias are spasmodic torticollis, in which there is sustained rotation of the head caused by involuntary contraction on one sternomastoid muscle, and writer's cramp, in which spasm of the muscles of the dominant hand and forearm occur whenever the patient attempts to write.

Response to treatment is often disappointing but a few patients are helped by high doses of anticholinergic drugs.

20. Multiple sclerosis

In temperate regions of the world, multiple sclerosis is one of the commoner chronic neurological diseases of young adults. Estimates of the prevalence in the UK suggest that more than 50 people per 100 000 have the disease. Women are affected slightly more frequently than men.

AETIOLOGY

Epidemiological studies of the geographical distribution of multiple sclerosis have provided several tantalizing clues about its aetiology. The occurrence of an epidemic of the disease in the Faroe Islands between 1943 and 1960 is one line of evidence that suggests the involvement of a transmissible agent. Almost all the cases of multiple sclerosis came from parts of the islands where British soldiers had been billeted during the military occupation of the island during the Second World War. It is conjectured that the soldiers introduced the causative agent, but so far the nature of the agent has not been identified.

Studies of the incidence of the disease in people who have migrated from a country where rates of multiple sclerosis are high to a place where the disease is rare suggest that an environmental agent acting in childhood is important. The rate of multiple sclerosis in those who migrated as children is similar to that of the host country. In contrast, the rate of disease amongst those who migrated in adult life is the same as that of the country from which they came.

There is strong evidence, too, that susceptibility to multiple sclerosis is genetically determined. The concordance rate for multiple sclerosis is higher in monozygotic twins than in dizygotic twins and, in some populations at least, the disease is associated with certain HLA subgroups.

Animal models of multiple sclerosis can be produced in both guinea pigs and monkeys by inoculating them with CNS tissue extracts. This fact, together with the abnormal immunoglobulins found in the CSF of some patients and the presence of lymphocytes and macrophages in the lesions of multiple sclerosis, has led to the conclusion that altered immunity is involved in the pathogenesis.

It seems unlikely that multiple sclerosis will turn out to have a single cause. Development of the disease probably requires the interaction of one or more, as yet unidentified, environmental agents in a genetically susceptible individual.

PATHOLOGY

Multiple sclerosis is a disease of the myelin of the central nervous system. The peripheral nerves are not affected. The pathological hallmark is the plaque of demyelination. In the early stages the plaque consists of an inflammatory cell infiltrate concentrated around small venules. Destruction of myelin occurs within and at the edge of the plaque and the surrounding area becomes oedematous. Later there is proliferation of glial cells. The areas of the central nervous system most frequently affected by plaque formation are the optic nerves, periventricular white matter within the cerebral hemispheres, the brain stem and the cervical spinal cord.

CLINICAL FEATURES

The disease usually starts in early adult life. It is rare before puberty or after the age of 50. In younger patients the disease usually follows a relapsing and remitting course. The acute appearance of neurological symptoms and disability is followed by a gradual complete or nearly complete recovery. Subsequent attacks occur at intervals varying from a few weeks to many years but the degree of recovery from later relapses is often less complete. When the disease develops for the first time in older patients it is more likely to pursue a slowly progressive course without apparent fluctuations in disease activity.

The speed of progression of the disease and the disability that results vary widely between patients. Occasionally, definite pathological changes of multiple sclerosis are found at autopsy in patients who have never had symptoms or shown signs of neurological disease. At the other extreme, a small proportion of cases experience a rapid deterioration leading to severe disability or even death within a few months of the onset of the first symptoms. Long-term follow-up studies have shown that, for the majority of patients, multiple sclerosis is a more benign disease than is generally recognized. About 75% of patients will still be alive 25 years after diagnosis and the majority of these will still be ambulant.

Symptoms at the onset of multiple sclerosis

No myelinated pathway in the central nervous system is immune from plaque formation so that the symptoms and signs of the disease are very variable.

Weakness in one arm or in one leg (monoparesis) or of both legs (paraparesis) is common as a first presentation of multiple sclerosis. The weakness is usually pyramidally distributed and other signs of corticospinal tract dysfunction—increased tendon reflexes and extensor plantar responses—are found on examination.

The dorsal columns in the cervical part of the spinal cord are frequently a site of plaque formation. The resulting loss of proprioceptive sensation may be extremely disabling. Patients describe an affected limb as useless even though there is no loss of muscle power. Lhermitte's sign—a sudden electric shock-like sensation shooting down the spine and into the arms or legs when the patient flexes his neck—is frequently present with cervical cord demyelinating lesions.

Involvement of the spinothalamic system often causes unpleasant paraesthesiae, for example, feelings of burning or of cold water running over the skin, as well as loss of pain and temperature sensation.

Sudden loss of visual acuity due to a plaque of demyelination in the optic nerve is known as *optic neuritis* or *retrobulbar neuritis*. The loss of visual acuity may be preceded by pain in or behind the eye, which is often exacerbated by eye movement. Central vision may be reduced to 6/60 or even lower, though the peripheral part of the visual field is often not affected. In the acute stages of optic neuritis the pupil of the affected eye is often slightly dilated and the pupillary light reflex is impaired. Recovery usually takes place slowly over a few weeks and visual acuity may return to normal. Some patients report a persisting abnormality in colour perception in that intense colours appear to be faded. Repeated attacks of optic neuritis cause optic atrophy. Visual acuity is permanently reduced and pallor of the optic disc is visible with an ophthalmoscope.

If the plaque of demyelination is situated immediately behind the head of the optic nerve the optic disc swells and mimics the appearances of papilloedema. This rarely causes diagnostic difficulty because swelling of the optic disc as a result of optic neuritis is always associated with profound loss of visual acuity. In cases of papilloedema from raised intracranial pressure visual acuity is usually preserved. More frequently the plaque is situated posteriorly in the optic nerve and the optic disc retains its normal appearance.

Subclinical attacks of optic neuritis also occur. It is common to find pallor of the optic disc in a patient with multiple sclerosis who gives no history of visual disturbance.

Other signs and symptoms typical of multiple sclerosis

No single clinical sign is pathognomonic of multiple sclerosis, but an internuclear ophthalmoplegia or ataxic nystagmus in a young person is very rarely caused by other diseases. Cerebellar signs—ataxia, dysarthria and nystagmus—are common and reflect demyelination in the cerebellar connections. Many patients suffer disturbance of sphincter control. The abdominal reflexes are usually lost early in the course of the disease. Changes of affect, which may be either depression or euphoria, are frequently seen, but true psychosis or dementia is rare. Epilepsy in patients with multiple sclerosis is uncommon but by no means unknown.

Diagnosis and investigations

The diagnosis of multiple sclerosis is based on finding evidence from the history and clinical examination of lesions in two or more parts of the central nervous system. The diagnosis becomes more certain if there have been several distinct episodes of neurological disturbance. Objective abnormalities of neurological function need to be present for a definite diagnosis to be made.

No laboratory test is diagnostic by itself but the following investigations may be helpful:

Visual evoked potentials

Abnormality of the visual evoked potential is a sensitive but non-specific indicator of damage in the visual pathway. The value of this test in multiple sclerosis is that it may demonstrate the presence of subclinical involvement of the optic nerve in a patient who gives no history of optic neuritis and who has apparently normal visual function.

CT scanning

A CT scan may show low density areas, often in a periventricular distribution, which represent plaques of demyelination. Magnetic resonance imaging is a more sensitive way of demonstrating plaques, but this technique is not yet widely available.

Examination of the CSF

Abnormalities in the CSF are present in a substantial proportion of patients with multiple sclerosis. Typically, there is a small increase in cell count and an increased fraction of γ-globulin. Electrophoresis of CSF will demonstrate the presence of oligoclonal immunoglobulin bands in the majority of cases.

TREATMENT

The history of specific treatments for multiple sclerosis is a sad story of the enthusiastic adoption and subsequent discarding of unproven remedies. Various diets, dietary supplements, immunosuppressive regimens, treatments intended to stimulate the immune response, and bizarre aberrations such as snake venom injections and scorpion bites have all been advocated at one time or another. Very few, until recently, have been tested in properly controlled clinical trials. So far, no treatment that has been subjected to careful evaluation has clearly been shown to be of benefit.

Treatment for sufferers from multiple sclerosis is symptomatic and supportive. Because sphincter control is often impaired, incontinence and urinary tract infections are common problems. Anticholinergics may help some patients with urge incontinence but they are of limited value. Antibiotics are required for urinary tract infections.

Spasticity can be controlled with baclofen. Careful adjustment of dose is necessary; reduction in spasticity may increase disability because it unmasks weakness.

Short courses of physiotherapy are useful in restoring mobility and in helping a patient regain confidence, especially after a relapse.

An occupational therapist may be able to suggest modifications to the patient's home which can be of enormous benefit in helping a disabled patient to cope with the difficulties of everyday living.

21. Peripheral neuropathy

Disorder of peripheral nerves are classified by their anatomical distribution into *mononeuropathies*, where only one peripheral nerve is affected; *multiple mononeuropathies*, an apparently contradictory term which indicates disease affecting several peripheral nerves simultaneously; *polyneuropathies*, in which the function of all peripheral nerves is disordered and *plexopathies*, where the whole or part of a nerve plexus is affected.

MONONEUROPATHY

The commonest causes of lesions of a single peripheral nerve are trauma and compression.

Trauma

Traumatic damage to a peripheral nerve severe enough to interrupt axonal continuity causes complete loss of motor and sensory function in the distribution of that nerve. Paralysis and wasting of muscles occurs and tendon reflexes are lost. There is complete cutaneous anaesthesia and, if the peripheral nerve carries autonomic fibres, there is also loss of sweating and disturbance of vasomotor function.

The prognosis for recovery after traumatic damage to a peripheral nerve depends on the nature of the injury. Complete anatomical division of the nerve results in degeneration of the distal part of the axons. The supporting connective tissue skeleton of the nerve is disrupted and, when regeneration begins, axon sprouts growing out from the proximal end are unlikely to make contact with the distal part of the nerve. The chances of any functional recovery are poor. Crushing injuries that leave the supporting skeleton of the nerve intact carry a better prognosis because axons can regenerate along their previous paths. Recovery is always slow because axons regrow at a rate of only a few millimetres each day.

Accurate diagnosis of traumatic peripheral nerve injuries depends on a careful clinical examination of muscle strength, tendon reflexes and cutaneous sensation. The short booklet *Aids to the Examination of the Peripheral Nervous System* (see Further Reading) is recommended to those who find it difficult to remember the details of the anatomy of the peripheral nervous system.

Compression

Local compression causes mechanical disruption of myelin sheaths at the point where pressure is exerted and block of conduction over a short segment of the nerve. Axonal damage and distal degeneration only occurs if pressure is exerted for a prolonged period. Recovery of function is usually rapid, beginning within a few days, and it is often complete after 6–8 weeks. When compression has been prolonged and axonal degeneration has taken place, recovery is much slower and less complete because it depends on the regrowth of axons from the proximal side of the lesion.

Large diameter nerve fibres resist pressure less well than small diameter fibres so that in compressive nerve lesions motor and proprioceptive function tend to be most severely affected. Although the patient may complain of paraesthesia and numbness, clinical examination of the modalities of touch, temperature and pain rarely reveal any major abnormality.

Some peripheral nerves are especially vulnerable to compression because they run superficially or over a bony prominence. Commonly occurring compressive mononeuropathies are described below.

Median nerve

Carpal tunnel syndrome, caused by the entrapment of the median nerve at the wrist as it passes under the flexor retinaculum, is one of the commonest compressive mononeuropathies. The syndrome occurs more frequently in women than men and is especially common during pregnancy. It may also be related to occupation (typists, seamstresses, slaters and others who operate tools which require repeated flexing of the wrist) or systemic disease (hypothyroidism, rheumatoid arthritis, acromegaly). Painful paraesthesiae, often worst at night, affect the hand. In addition, there may be sensory loss in the cutaneous distribution of the median nerve in the hand (the flexor aspect of the thumb, index, middle and radial half of the ring fingers and the radial half of the palm) and weakness and wasting of the muscles of the thenar eminence innervated by the median nerve (abductor pollicis brevis, flexor pollicis and opponens pollicis). Abductor pollicis brevis is usually the most severely affected muscle.

Injection of hydrocortisone directly into the carpal tunnel may give relief of symptom, but often the benefit is only temporary. The most effective treatment is surgical division of the flexor retinaculum.

Ulnar nerve

Weakness of the intrinsic muscles of the hand that spares the thenar eminence, together with sensory loss over the lateral border of the hand are the features of ulnar nerve lesions. The common site of compression is at the elbow where the nerve passes under the medial epicondyle. Deformity of the elbow joint as a result of arthritis or fracture predisposes to ulnar nerve compression.

Radial nerve

This nerve is vulnerable to compression against the shaft of the humerus. Compressive radial nerve lesions are known as Saturday night palsy because a common reason for the condition is supposed to be falling asleep drunk with the arm hanging over the back of a chair. There is weakness of the extensors of the wrist and fingers and sensory loss over the radial side of the dorsum of the hand.

Common peroneal nerve

Damage may occur to this nerve at the point where it winds around the head of the fibula. Foot drop and sensory loss over the lateral part of the shin and dorsum of the foot are the main clinical features. Patients with badly fitting below-knee plaster casts are at risk of compressing this nerve.

Lateral cutaneous nerve of the thigh

Meralgia paraesthetica is the term given to a syndrome of pain and numbness over the anterolateral thigh that results from compression of the lateral cutaneous nerve of the thigh as it passes under the inguinal ligament.

Posterior tibial nerve

The medial plantar branch of the posterior tibial nerve may be compressed as it passes under the flexor retinaculum of the foot just behind the medial malleolus. Symptoms of pain and numbness are localized to the medial side of the sole of the foot. Surgical decompression of the nerve by division of the retinaculum is the definitive treatment.

CRANIAL MONONEUROPATHIES

Bell's palsy is an idiopathic mononeuropathy of the facial nerve caused by swelling of the nerve within the bony confines of the facial canal. The condition presents with rapid onset of a lower motor neurone type of facial palsy. Frequently the facial weakness is preceded by pain in and behind the ear. Taste on the ipsilateral side of the tongue is often affected and, if the nerve is involved proximally, before the branch to stapedius is given off, hyperacusis may be present. The causes of facial palsy are considered in more detail in Chapter 28.

Mononeuropathies of the oculomotor (III), trochlear (IV) or abducens (VI) nerve may occur as a result of ischaemia or infarction of the nerve trunk. The usual presentation is of sudden onset of painless diplopia in an elderly patient. Diabetes and hypertension are common underlying causes but a careful search for other intracranial pathology is required before diagnosing an oculomotor nerve palsy as due to ischaemic mononeuropathy.

MULTIPLE MONONEUROPATHY

Loss of function in several peripheral nerves at the same time may occur as a complication of a number of systemic diseases:

1. Diabetes mellitus
2. Polyarteritis nodosa
3. Other connective tissue diseases

4. Sarcoidosis
5. Neurofibromatosis.

The underlying pathology in diabetes, polyarteritis nodosa and the other connective tissue diseases is ischaemia of the nerve trunk secondary to thrombosis of the vasa nervorum. In sarcoidosis the neuropathy is caused by the presence of sarcoid granulomata within the peripheral nerve. In neurofibromatosis, the nerves are directly affected by multiple tumours.

The clinical features of multiple mononeuropathy are of muscle weakness and wasting and sensory loss in the distribution of the affected nerves.

POLYNEUROPATHY

A number of drugs, toxins, infections and metabolic disorders have an adverse effect on the function of peripheral nerves and may produce a polyneuropathy (Table 21.1). Depending on the cause,

Table 21.1   Causes of polyneuropathy

Motor neuropathies	Guillain-Barré syndrome Drugs: gold 　　　　dapsone Lead poisoning Exposure to n-hexane Diphtheria Acute intermittent porphyria
Sensory polyneuropathies	Drugs: isoniazid 　　　　phenytoin Uraemia Leprosy
Mixed polyneuropathies	Diabetes mellitus Alcohol Drugs: vincristine 　　　　nitrofurantoin 　　　　perhexiline 　　　　chlorambucil Vitamin deficiency: thiamine 　　　　　　　vitamin B_{12} Hereditary polyneuropathies Paraneoplastic complication of malignant disease Connective tissue diseases Uraemia Exposure to acrylamide
Autonomic neuropathy	Diabetes mellitus Primary amyloidosis

the pathology may be either demyelination or axonal degeneration, or a combination of the two. Sensory, motor and autonomic function are affected to a different extent by different agents. Careful evaluation of the pathology and the type of nerve fibre predominantly affected helps to narrow down the search for the underlying cause.

Clinical features

Diseases which affect peripheral nerves generally have their most marked effects on nerve cells with the longest axons. Symptoms and signs, therefore, tend to be most prominent in the distal parts of the limbs. The motor signs of polyneuropathy are distal weakness and muscle wasting. Tendon reflexes are reduced or absent. The ankle jerks are usually the first to disappear. Sensory symptoms of paraethesia and numbness are accompanied by signs of impaired sensation to modalities of joint position, vibration, touch, temperature and pain. The distal distribution of sensory disturbance is commonly described as 'glove and stocking' sensory loss. Common autonomic features are impotence, postural hypotension, abnormalities of sweating, cardiac arrhythmias and disturbance of bladder function.

Diagnosis and investigations

Diagnosing the presence of peripheral neuropathy is usually straightforward but finding the underlying cause is often much harder. Important evidence may be obtained from a thorough history of the drugs that the patient has been taking, from an occupational history or from a full family history of neurological disease. A search for endocrine, connective tissue, neoplastic and metabolic diseases may be necessary. Nerve conductive studies, described in Chapter 14, confirm the diagnosis of polyneuropathy and are valuable in distinguishing neuropathies caused by axonal damage from those caused by demyelination. Biopsy of a peripheral sensory nerve, usually the sural nerve, is sometimes carried out in an attempt to advance the diagnosis in peripheral neuropathies whose cause is obscure.

Metabolic and toxic causes of polyneuropathy

Diabetes mellitus

A symmetrical, distal, predominantly sensory polyneuropathy is present in a high proportion of long-standing diabetics. In many cases it is asymptomatic and revealed only at clinical examination by the absence of ankle jerks and reduction in distal sensation.

In a smaller proportion, the neuropathy is symptomatic. Peripheral sensory loss may result in ulceration and trophic changes in the feet and in the formation of Charcot joints. Sometimes the neuropathy is painful; unpleasant paraesthesiae, often burning in nature, are present in the feet and legs.

Diabetic peripheral neuropathy frequently involves the autonomic fibres causing impotence, abnormalities of sweating, postural hypotension and an increase in resting heart rate.

Diabetic amyotrophy is a neuropathic complication of diabetes which should really be included under the heading of multiple mononeuropathy or plexopathy. It is a painful condition resulting from infarction of parts of the lumbosacral plexus or the femoral nerve itself. Profound wasting and weakness of the quadriceps develops over a short time, in association with pain over the anterior and medial part of the thigh, sometimes extending down into the calf.

Treatment of all forms of diabetic peripheral neuropathy is directed at improving glycaemic control. Recovery is often limited and may be delayed for many months.

Uraemia

A symmetrical, mainly sensory, polyneuropathy is present in many cases of chronic renal failure.

Vitamin deficiency

Deficiency of vitamin B_{12} causes a sensory neuropathy, mainly affecting large diameter fibres. There are often associated features of a central neuropathy — subacute combined degeneration of the spinal cord (see Ch.24).

In the developing world, deficiency of vitamin B_1 (thiamine) is a common cause of polyneuropathy. In the UK, thiamine deficiency is almost entirely restricted to chronic alcoholics. There are symptoms of a painful motor and sensory peripheral neuropathy. The condition responds to treatment with thiamine.

Drugs

A list of drugs which are known to cause peripheral neuropathy is included in Table 21.1. Most cause a fairly mild distal sensory disturbance. Dapsone is an exception in affecting only motor fibres.

Hereditary polyneuropathy

A number of inherited disorders of peripheral nerves exist. The most important is Charcot-Marie-Tooth disease, which is also known as peroneal muscular atrophy and as hereditary motor and sensory neuropathy, often abbreviated to HMSN. It is most commonly inherited as a dominant trait but recessive forms also exist.

Clinical features

There is a very slowly progressive distal weakness with muscle wasting. The appearance of the first symptoms is often delayed into adult life. The distal wasting produces a characteristic appearance of the lower limbs which resemble inverted champagne bottles. Pes cavus is a common feature and there is wasting of the intrinsic muscles of the hand. Because of foot drop the patient walks with a high stepping gait. Motor symptoms predominate but there is also an accompanying distal sensory loss. In some cases the peripheral nerves are thickened and may be palpable. Disability is usually slight and life expectancy is not affected.

Treatment

Treatment is symptomatic. Fitting shoes with toe-spring splints improves gait. Patients must be warned to take special care of their feet because the distal sensory loss makes them vulnerable to minor trauma.

Paraneoplastic neuropathy

Sensory polyneuropathy is an unusual paraneoplastic complication of several neoplasms, bronchogenic carcinoma being the commonest. The neuropathy may be severe enough to cause sensory ataxia. Occasionally neuropathic symptoms may precede the appearance of the underlying neoplasm by several years.

Guillain-Barré syndrome

This is an immunologically mediated condition in which

demyelination, starting in nerve roots and subsequently extending into peripheral nerves, causes a subacute, mainly motor polyneuropathy.

Clinical features

The first symptoms are often sensory, consisting of distal paraesthesia of the feet and hands. Next, muscle weakness develops, usually starting distally in the limbs and ascending to involve all limb segments and sometimes the facial and respiratory musculature too, over the course of a few days. A proportion of cases give a history of a preceding viral infection. The severity of the condition is very variable, but in about 10% of cases weakness is so profound and widespread that ventilation is required. Tendon reflexes are invariably lost. Despite the early sensory symptoms, sensory loss may be difficult to demonstrate clinically. A variant of the condition exists in which cranial nerves are predominantly affected. Weakness is maximal within 2−3 weeks of the onset of neurological symptoms. Recovery is slow and it is often many months before full strength is regained. There is a small but significant mortality.

Investigations

The clinical diagnosis is confirmed by measurement of nerve conduction velocities which are usually profoundly slowed. Examination of the CSF demonstrates a greatly raised protein concentration in the absence of a corresponding increase in the cell count.

Treatment

The greatest hazard to the patient is respiratory failure. Respiratory function should be monitored by repeated measurement of vital capacity and artificial ventilation started before respiratory failure develops. In the most severely affected patients ventilation may be required for prolonged periods.

Physiotherapy is essential to prevent the development of contractures and to maintain mobility of joints.

Plasmapheresis, if performed early during the course of the disease, may be of value, but its place is controversial.

Amyloidosis

Symptoms of a sensory and autonomic peripheral neuropathy are present in about 15% of patients with primary amyloidosis. Rarely, neuropathic symptoms occur with amyloidosis secondary to multiple myeloma and paraproteinaemia. An unusual feature is the predominance of symptoms of autonomic dysfunction.

PLEXOPATHY

Thoracic outlet syndromes

The presence of a cervical rib or a fibrous band originating from the transverse process of the 7th cervical vertebra may compress the lower part of the brachial plexus. Symptoms are of pain in the distribution of the C8 and T1 dermatomes and weakness of the small muscle of the hand. Surgical removal of the cervical rib or division of the fibrous band is necessary when symptoms are severe.

Brachial neuritis

This condition, also known as neuralgic amyotrophy, starts with severe pain in the shoulder and upper arm. The pain subsides within a few days but is followed by the development of weakness and muscle wasting in a patchy, usually proximal distribution. Tendon reflexes in the affected arm are often lost and there may be an accompanying sensory deficit.

Recovery is slow and may be incomplete. Rarely, the condition occurs bilaterally.

The aetiology is unknown, but a recent observation suggests that it may follow parvovirus infection.

Trauma

Severe trauma to the shoulder, if it involves distraction of the arm, may result in damage to the brachial plexus. The upper roots tend to bear the brunt of the injury. Recovery is very limited and the patient may be left with a permanently anaesthetic and paralysed arm.

Radiation

Damage to the upper roots of the brachial plexus causing weakness and atrophy of the muscles of the shoulder and upper arm is an occasional sequel to radiation treatment given for carcinoma of the breast.

Malignant infiltration

Neoplastic infiltration, most commonly by an apically situated carcinoma of the lung, may involve the lower roots of the plexus. The clinical features are distal weakness and muscle wasting and sensory loss in the hand and forearm.

22. Disorders of skeletal muscle

The term muscular dystrophy is generally used to mean an inherited degenerative disorder of muscle. This is in contrast to myopathies and inflammatory disorders of muscle, which are either acquired or secondary to some other disease process. There are also a number of rare muscle diseases which result from a specific defect in one of the pathways of energy metabolism. The cause of most of these is unknown, and may, in some cases, be genetic.

In adults, the common presenting symptoms of muscle disease are weakness and muscle wasting. In children, muscle disease is more likely to present as a failure to reach normal developmental milestones at the expected age. Important aspects to consider in the clinical history are age of onset of symptoms, whether it is the proximal or distal muscles that are mainly affected, whether the bulbar, facial and sternomastoid muscles are also involved and whether there is a family history of muscle disease.

MUSCULAR DYSTROPHIES

Duchenne muscular dystrophy

This condition is inherited as an X-linked recessive gene. Cases of the disease are therefore restricted to males with females being carriers. On average, half the sons born to a woman who carries the gene will be affected and half the daughters will be carriers.

The disease usually presents at the age of 3 or 4 years in a child who, until that time, has developed normally. The first muscles to be affected are those of the hip girdle and the earliest symptoms are of difficulty in getting up from the ground and in climbing stairs. The weakness spreads slowly to all muscle groups and by the age of 10 most patients are unable to walk. In the earlier stages the calf muscles, and sometimes quadriceps too, become enlarged. This is partly the result of fatty infiltration and partly because of true hypertrophy of the remaining muscle fibres. Progressive muscular wasting leads to skeletal deformity and contractures. Cardiomyopathy invariably accompanies the disease. Few cases survive beyond the age of 20 years. Death is often due to respiratory infection or cardiac failure.

A similar, but much more benign condition known as Becker dystrophy occurs. It is also inherited as an X-linked gene. The age of onset is later and the rate of deterioration is much slower.

Measurement of plasma concentrations of the muscle enzyme creatine kinase allows detection of the majority of female carriers of the defective gene and is helpful in genetic counselling of affected families.

Facioscapulohumeral muscular dystrophy

This disorder is inherited as an autosomal dominant trait. The disease becomes symptomatic in adolescence with weakness of the muscles of the shoulder girdle and face. Patients have a characteristic pouting expression and, when examined, have striking winging of the scapulae. The disease is only very slowly progressive and few patients become severely disabled.

Dystrophia myotonica

This is the commonest of the muscular dystrophies. It, too, is inherited as an autosomal dominant trait. The condition usually presents between the ages of 20 and 50 years with predominantly distal weakness in arms and legs. Patients complain of tripping up and falling easily and of weakness of grip. They have a typical scrawny facial appearance with ptosis, wasting of masseters, temporalis and sternomastoids (Fig. 22.1). Affected males show frontal balding. The disease is associated with premature cataract formation, cardiomyopathy, disturbance of cardiac conduction and gonadal atrophy.

Myotonia refers to the phenomenon of persistence of active muscle contraction after voluntary effort has ceased. It is due to an abnormality of the membrane of the muscle fibre and can be demonstrated electromyographically as a continuing discharge of action potentials. Myotonia can be seen if the patient is asked to clench his fist and then to spread his fingers; several seconds may

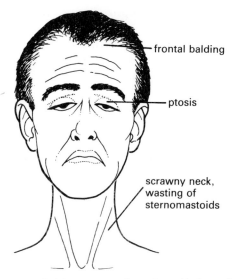

Fig. 22.1 The typical facial appearance of a patient with dystrophia myotonica.

elapse before the fingers are fully extended. This feature may be dramatic, especially if the patient is examined in a cold room, but from the patient's point of view the disabling feature of the disease is usually muscle weakness rather than myotonia. Few activities, other than playing a musical instrument, throwing a dart at a dartboard, or firing an automatic weapon, demand great rapidity of muscle relaxation.

ENDOCRINE MYOPATHIES

In adults, endocrine disorders are one of the commonest causes of proximal myopathy. Investigations of thyroid and adrenal function should always be carried out. Symptoms of muscle weakness respond to treatment of the underlying disease.

Thyrotoxicosis

Proximal myopathy, predominantly affecting the shoulder girdle and proximal arm muscles, is commonly found in patients with thyrotoxicosis. In elderly hyperthyroid women the classical symptoms of weight loss, heat intolerance and irritability are notoriously absent and myopathy may be the presenting symptom.

In a proportion of cases of Graves' disease, infiltration of the external ocular muscles with fat and inflammatory cells causes ophthalmoplegia and exophthalmos.

Hypothyroidism

Stiffness and muscle cramps are common in hypothyroidism though significant weakness is unusual. Speed of muscle relaxation is slowed because of a reduction in the rate of uncoupling of Actinomyosin cross-bridges. This is sometimes noticeable as a short but definite delay in the onset of relaxation during clinical examination of tendon reflexes.

Cushing's syndrome

Corticosteroids are anabolic and loss of muscle mass is a feature of Cushing's syndrome and an iatrogenic complication of prolonged steroid treatment. Weakness mainly affects the proximal muscles.

METABOLIC MYOPATHIES

Disorders of glycogenolysis

Glycogen is an important energy substrate for muscle. If the enzyme myophosphorylase is deficient, glucose cannot be liberated from muscle glycogen stores and metabolized to produce ATP. Myophosphorylase deficiency causes a syndrome of severe muscular pain and stiffness precipitated by moderate exercise. The condition can be diagnosed by showing that blood lactate concentrations fail to rise after exercise. This condition, known as McArdle's syndrome, is extremely rare but interesting because its biochemistry is so well understood. A few other, even rarer, enzyme deficiencies exist in which there is defective utilization of glycogen.

Mitochondrial disorders

Mitochondrial myopathy is a term used to cover a variety of rare metabolic disorders in which there is either defective transport of energy substrate into mitochondria or defective energy metabolism within the organelle. In some cases the myopathy is part of a generalized disease which includes retinal and cerebellar degeneration and cardiomyopathy. Histochemically, mitochondrial myopathies are characterized by an abnormality of type 1 fibres known as ragged red fibres. Biochemical techniques have identified a number of specific enzyme deficiences associated with the histological abnormalities.

POLYMYOSITIS

This term covers an aetiologically heterogeneous group of inflammatory muscle disorders which are characterized by acute or subacute onset of weakness, sometimes in association with muscle pain and tenderness, dysphagia and facial and respiratory weakness. In addition, inflammatory skin changes may be present; these consist of a bluish violet erythema around the eyes and in the nail beds and an erythematous rash on the extensor surfaces of the limbs. When skin lesions are present the disorder is known as *dermatomyositis*.

In about a third of cases polymyositis is part of a connective tissue disease syndrome such as systemic lupus erythematosus or systemic sclerosis. In older people, particularly older men, dermatomyositis can be a manifestation of malignancy. The tumour is often occult at the time of presentation with dermatomyositis.

Plasma concentrations of creatine kinase are elevated and the ESR may be raised. Electromyography is often helpful in confirming the diagnosis. Muscle biopsy shows necrotic muscle fibres and a patchy infiltration of inflammatory cells.

Treatment with steroids is usually effective. High doses, of up to 120 mg prednisolone per day, may be needed and immunosuppressant drugs are often required in addition. Some cases fail to respond and, as a last resort, whole body irradiation may be tried. The prognosis for remission is best in children and young adults. In patients who develop polymyositis in middle age the disease often becomes chronic.

POLYMYALGIA RHEUMATICA

This is a syndrome found in elderly patients, in which there is widespread muscular stiffness and pain, particularly of the shoulder and hip girdles. Muscles are often tender but actual weakness is absent. There is usually a systemic upset with malaise and a very high ESR. In some cases polymyalgia is associated with giant cell arteritis (see Ch. 29) but otherwise the cause is unknown. It responds dramatically to treatment with steroids.

INVESTIGATION OF MUSCLE DISEASE

Creatine kinase

Plasma concentrations of the muscle enzyme creatine kinase are often elevated in muscle disease because of leakage of the enzyme from damaged and necrotic muscle fibres. Levels of creatine kinase depend on the rate of destruction of muscle fibres and tend to be higher in inflammatory disorders of muscle than in chronic metabolic myopathies or muscular dystrophies.

Electromyography

Electrophysiological studies of muscle are valuable in confirming a diagnosis of primary muscle disease and in distinguishing muscle weakness caused by myopathy from weakness resulting from disease of peripheral nerves. Electromyographic features are rarely specific for particular muscle diseases, although the myotonic discharges of dystrophia myotonica are an exception.

Muscle biopsy

Accurate diagnosis of muscle disease, particularly those caused by specific disorders of metabolism, usually requires histological examination of a muscle biopsy supplemented by electron microscopy and histochemical and biochemical techniques.

23. Myasthenia gravis

Myasthenia gravis is a chronic disease characterized by muscle weakness and a great exaggeration of the normal fatigue that follows sustained muscular contraction. The frequent association of this disease with autoimmune disorders, in particular thyrotoxicosis, was an important clue in unravelling its pathogenesis. It is now known that, in the vast majority of cases, a circulating IgG globulin directed at the acetyl choline receptor on the muscle endplate is present. Although normal quantities of acetyl choline are released from the motor nerve terminal, neuromuscular transmission fails because of the immunologically mediated destruction of receptor sites on the postsynaptic membrane.

In most patients the disease is associated with hyperplasia of the thymus but in a small proportion, about 15%, a thymoma is present. The prognosis is much poorer in the latter group because the tumour tends to recur after surgical removal.

CLINICAL FEATURES

Women are affected twice as often as men. The disease is rare before adult life and the incidence is highest between the ages of 20 to 40 years. Weakness and fatiguability are often restricted to particular groups of muscles. External ocular, facial and bulbar muscles are the most frequently involved, but symptoms in the muscles of the limbs and axial skeleton are not uncommon. At presentation the initial symptoms and signs are confined to the external ocular muscles in about 20% of patients but half of these will eventually progress to generalized myasthenia.

Myasthenia may affect any combination of external ocular muscles and the presence of an eye movement disorder which cannot be explained by a single cranial nerve palsy or a disorder of conjugate gaze should always suggest this diagnosis. Myasthenic weakness of the face is manifested by ptosis, weakness of eye closure and a transverse smile in which the corners of the mouth fail to turn up. Involvement of bulbar muscles causes dysphonia, dysarthria and dysphagia. The speech of a myasthenic patient is normal at the beginning of a sentence but progressively becomes quieter and slurred. Weakness of the palate gives the voice a nasal quality.

The second word of the name of the disease, *gravis*, should not be forgotten. A small subgroup of patients present with, or rapidly progress to, severe disease in which weakness of bulbar and respiratory musculature may be profound enough to be life threatening.

Examination will confirm the presence of weakness and of easy fatiguability. Tendon reflexes are usually brisk, although they may disappear if tested repeatedly. Muscle wasting is sometimes present in myasthenia but only as a late complication of severe disease.

Investigations

The Tensilon test

Intravenous injection of the short-acting cholinesterase inhibitor edrophonium (Tensilon) causes a transient increase in the amount of acetyl choline present at the neuromuscular junction and facilitates neuromuscular transmission. The test is only useful if some objective signs of muscle weakness are present at the time the test is performed. Ten millilitres of edrophonium should be given; 2 ml are injected and, providing no adverse effects occur, the remaining 8 ml are injected as a bolus 1 minute later. A transient increase in muscle strength, or decrease in diplopia following the injection, is strong evidence in favour of a diagnosis of myasthenia.

Electromyography

In normal subjects repetitive stimulation of a motor nerve causes only slight reduction in the amplitude of the muscle action potential up to rates of 30 per second. In myasthenics there is a progressive decline in the amplitude of the action potential. It is important to select a symptomatic muscle for this test.

Anti-ACh receptor antibody

Circulating antibodies to the acetyl choline receptor can be detected by a radioimmunoassay technique in about 90% of patients with generalized myasthenia and about 70% of patients with purely ocular disease.

Computerized tomography of the anterior mediastinum

This should be carried out to determine if a thymoma is present.

TREATMENT

Anticholinesterase drugs

Drug treatment with long-acting anticholinesterases (neostigmine and pyridostigmine) often alleviates symptoms dramatically. Great care must be taken to avoid overdosage. Too high a dose causes accumulation of acetyl choline at the neuromuscular junction, with depolarization block of neuromuscular transmission and a worsening of muscle weakness. Difficulties in judging the optimum dosage arise because a dose of anticholinesterase that is inadequate for one muscle group may be excessive for another. Cramping abdominal pain, the result of cholinergic stimulation of the gastrointestinal tract, is a frequent side-effect of anticholinesterase treatment. Propantheline or atropine is useful in counteracting these symptoms.

Immunosuppression

Immunosuppression with high doses of steroids, sometimes in combination with azathioprine, is a useful treatment in cases which fail to respond adequately to treatment with anticholinergics alone. There is often a transient exacerbation of myasthenic weakness following the introduction of steroids and close supervision in the early stages of steroid treatment is essential.

Plasmapheresis, with the aim of removing the circulating antibody, is sometimes tried but the clinical response is unpredictable and usually short-lived. This treatment is usually reserved for the treatment of a myasthenic crisis.

Thymectomy

Thymectomy may induce a prolonged remission, or at least a very significant improvement in symptoms, especially if carried out early in the course of the disease. Except in cases of purely ocular myasthenia, or unless the perioperative risk is thought too high, this treatment is now usually recommended. The presence of a thymoma is a strong indication for surgery because these tumours are locally invasive.

Drugs to be avoided in myasthenia

Aminoglycoside antibiotics, e.g. gentamicin and streptomycin, possess a minor degree of curare-like activity and are contraindicated in myasthenia.

Penicillamine, used in the treatment of rheumatoid arthritis, is a rare cause of myasthenia. Anti-ACh receptor antibodies are usually present and symptoms may not remit even when the drug is withdrawn.

MYASTHENIC SYNDROME

This condition, also known as the Eaton-Lambert syndrome, is a uncommon paraneoplastic complication, usually of oat cell carcinoma of the lung. As in myasthenia gravis, the main symptoms are muscle weakness and fatiguability. However, unlike myasthenia gravis, it is the proximal limb muscles that are predominantly affected and involvement of ocular and bulbar muscles is exceptional. The pathology lies in a deficiency of the amount of acetyl choline released from the endings of motor nerves and not in any defect of the postsynaptic membrane. The condition does not respond to treatment with anticholinesterase drugs and the Tensilon test is negative. Guanidine, a drug which enhances the release of acetyl choline, may be an effective treatment and the symptoms may remit if the underlying tumour is removed surgically.

24. Diseases of the spinal cord

SPINAL CORD COMPRESSION

The spinal cord is enclosed within a rigid bony tube formed by the arches and bodies of the vertebrae. This anatomical arrangement, which is extremely successful in protecting the spinal cord from all but the most severe external trauma, carries the disadvantage that any expanding lesion situated inside the vertebral canal is bound to press upon and distort the spinal cord. Blood vessels supplying the cord are also vulnerable to compression and ischaemia may contribute to the damage. A list of causes of spinal cord compression is given in Table 24.1.

Acute spinal cord compression

Acute cord compression is almost always the result of traumatic spinal injury involving fracture and dislocation of the vertebral column. There is a sudden onset of paralysis and sensory loss below the level of the lesion and loss of sphincter control. Incomplete lesions need urgent radiological investigation to identify the site of instability. Internal fixation of unstable fractures and sur-

Table 24.1 Causes of spinal cord compression

Spinal trauma	Fracture/dislocation of the spine
Intervertebral disc disease	Acute cervical central disc prolapse Cervical spondylosis
Neoplasms	Extradural (usually metastatic from lung, breast, prostate, kidney or multiple myeloma) Extramedullary (neurofibroma, meningioma) Intramedullary (astrocytoma, ependymoma)
Extradural abscess	Pyogenic Tuberculous

gical decompression of the cord may be necessary to prevent further damage occurring. Little can be done to reverse the effects of complete cord transection. The care of a patient with acute paraplegia is discussed later in the chapter.

Progressive spinal cord compression

Progressive cord compression by an expanding lesion causes a more gradual sequence of symptoms. In the earliest stages motor symptoms usually predominate with the patient complaining of weak and stiff legs. Examination reveals signs of corticospinal tract dysfunction with a pyramidally distributed weakness, spasticity, increased tendon reflexes and bilateral extensor plantar responses. As the underlying condition progresses sensory features become apparent. Paraesthesia and numbness start in the feet and gradually ascend to a sensory level corresponding to the spinal segment affected. Loss of bladder control is a late symptom and, unless decompression of the cord is undertaken urgently, the damage will be irreversible.

Causes of progressive spinal cord compression

Spinal neoplasms. Spinal tumours may arise extradurally, intradurally or within the substance of the cord itself.

Extradural tumours are almost always metastatic. Common sources are primaries in lung, breast, prostate or kidney and multiple myeloma. The prognosis is poor.

The common intradural tumours are neurofibromas and meningiomas. They are both slow-growing benign tumours and the prognosis after surgical removal is good.

Intramedullary tumours, i.e. tumours arising from within the spinal cord, are very uncommon. Most are benign astrocytomas or ependymomas. They are slow growing and progression of symptoms is gradual over several years.

Cervical spondylosis. Osteoarthritic changes in the cervical spine inevitably accompany ageing. Trauma to the neck tends to accelerate the degenerative process. In many people cervical spondylosis causes no more than pain and discomfort but in a few the combination of osteophyte formation, thickening of the ligamentum flavum and anterior bulging of the annulus fibrosus of the intervertebral disc reduces the internal dimensions of the cervical canal to the point where there is significant compression of the cervical spinal cord. Narrowing of the nerve root exit foramina may produce symptoms and signs of cervical root compression.

The clinical features are of a spastic paraparesis accompanied by lower motor neurone signs in the arms. Occasionally pain in the distribution of a cervical root or paraesthesia in the hands is present. Often there is no pain in the neck. The severity of symptoms and disability from cervical spondylosis varies widely between individuals. In milder cases, especially if they are elderly, full investigation by myelography may not be justified and conservative treatment with a cervical collar is all that is required. In more severe or progressive disease myelography is needed to confirm the diagnosis and identify the levels at which the compression is present. Surgical treatment by decompressive laminectomy or anterior fusion of the vertebral bodies usually arrests progression of symptoms, but it is rare for there to be much improvement.

Spinal abscess. An extradural pyogenic abscess caused by metastatic spread from a staphylococcal infective focus elsewhere in the body is a rare cause of rapid progressive spinal cord compression (see also Ch. 27).

Tuberculosis is now a rare cause of spinal abscess in the UK and is almost confined to the immigrant population.

Intervertebral disc prolapse. Acute prolapse of an intervertebral disc is very rare in the thoracic region but occasionally occurs, sometimes as a result of trauma, cervically. Central prolapse causes symptoms of cord compression. Lateral prolapse causes root compression with pain in the arm, motor weakness and sensory loss in the distribution of the affected root.

Investigations

Plain X-ray films of the spine may show bony changes or soft tissue shadows which hint strongly at the underlying diagnosis, but the definitive investigation in cases of progressive spinal cord compression is myelography. The changes in CSF hydrodynamics which follow the injection of contrast medium at myelography may precipitate an acute deterioration in the patient's condition and this investigation should only be undertaken in a neurosurgical centre where facilities for immediate laminectomy and decompression are available.

Treatment and prognosis

Early diagnosis of spinal cord compression caused by non-malignant lesions, followed by surgical intervention, particularly if carried out before bladder symptoms have developed, generally carries a good prognosis for recovery. However, if treatment is delayed until severe neurological deficit is present little improvement can be expected.

Cord compression which is the result of malignant disease carries a poor prognosis. Bony destruction by the tumour makes surgical intervention technically very difficult and radiotherapy is often preferable.

VITAMIN B_{12} MYELOPATHY (Subacute combined degeneration of the spinal cord)

Cyanocobalamin is an essential cofactor in steps of intermediary metabolism that involve the transfer of methyl groups. Large myelinated nerve fibres are especially vulnerable to deficiencies of this vitamin. The dorsal columns and corticospinal tracts of the spinal cord and large diameter fibres in peripheral nerves are most severely affected. In a few patients the optic nerves and the white matter of the cerebral hemispheres may also be involved.

The neurological consequences of vitamin B_{12} deficiency are usually, but not always, associated with pernicious anaemia. The commonest underlying cause of vitamin B_{12} deficiency is absence of intrinsic factor in association with gastric achlorhydria. Partial or total gastrectomy and diseases which affect the terminal ileum can also cause malabsorption of this vitamin.

Clinical features

The neurological symptoms and signs of vitamin B_{12} deficiency are due to the combined features of dysfunction of peripheral nerves and dorsal columns and corticospinal tracts of the spinal cord. The large fibre peripheral neuropathy causes distal paraesthesia, symmetrical sensory loss and loss of tendon reflexes (especially the ankle jerks). The involvement of the dorsal columns contributes to the loss of proprioceptive and vibration sensation and leads to a sensory ataxia. Dysfunction of the corticospinal tracts causes muscle weakness, which is most marked in the flexors of the lower limbs. Plantar responses are extensor. Disturbance of sphincter function is uncommon.

The speed of onset of symptoms is variable but the tempo is usually subacute rather than chronic. In addition to the neurological features there is usually evidence of a megaloblastic anaemia.

Investigations

The diagnosis is confirmed by measurement of serum vitamin B_{12} concentrations. Studies of vitamin B_{12} absorption are needed to determine the underlying cause of the deficiency.

Treatment

Frequent parenteral injections of vitamin B_{12} should be given as soon as the diagnosis is confirmed in order to restore tissue stores. Maintenance doses will be needed for the rest of the patient's life. Slow improvement in the symptoms of peripheral neuropathy may be expected, but little regeneration is possible in the spinal cord. Progression of the symptoms is arrested but, unless the disease has been diagnosed and treated early, some disability is likely to remain.

SYRINGOMYELIA

This term is derived from the Greek word syrinx, meaning pipe, and refers to a chronic condition of cavitation of the central part of the spinal cord. Very frequently, syringomyelia is found in association with developmental anomalies at the craniovertebral junction and it is thought that the central cavity of the cord is secondary to an abnormality in the outflow of CSF from the 4th ventricle. The cavity often extends longitudinally for most of the length of the cord and may reach rostrally into the medulla (syringobulbia). Dilatation is almost invariably maximal in the cervical region and most of the signs and symptoms are found in the upper limbs. The distortion of the spinal cord produced by the syrinx damages the decussating sensory nerve fibres of the spinothalamic tract, the cell bodies of the motor neurones in the anterior horn of the spinal grey matter and, to a lesser extent the descending fibres of the corticospinal tracts. Dorsal column function is relatively unaffected.

Clinical features

Syringomyelia is a chronic and slowly progressive condition. The

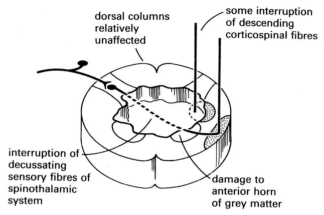

dorsal columns
relatively
unaffected

some interruption
of descending
corticospinal fibres

interruption of
decussating
sensory fibres of
spinothalamic
system

damage to
anterior horn
of grey matter

Fig. 24.1 The effects of a central lesion in the spinal cord.

onset of symptoms may occur at any age but is commonest in early adult life. The clinical features may be easily understood by reference to the anatomy of the lesion (Fig. 24.1).

Damage to the decussating spinothalamic fibres results in loss of pain and temperature sensation in the upper limbs and over the upper part of the thorax. Patients with syringomyelia often have burns, ulcers and wounds on their hands because loss of pain sensation robs them of the withdrawal reflex. Pain no longer protects against excessive forces applied to joints and traumatic osteoarthropathy (a Charcot joint) is often present at the shoulder or elbow. Examination reveals loss of sensation to pinprick and temperature but joint position, vibration and touch sensation are preserved. Loss of the sensory modalities of pain and temperature when proprioceptive and touch sensation are intact is known as *dissociated anaesthesia*.

Damage to anterior horn cells causes weakness and wasting of arm muscles; the small muscles of the hand are most affected. The monosynaptic reflex arc mediating the tendon reflex is disrupted and most patients with syringomyelia lack tendon reflexes in their upper limbs. Involvement of descending fibres in the corticospinal tracts is rarely severe but a minor degree of weakness and spasticity in the lower limbs is common.

Investigations

Confirmation of the clinical diagnosis may be obtained

radiographically by myelography. CT scanning of the cervical cord and craniovertebral junction after injection of contrast medium into the subarachnoid space may demonstrate the cavity itself. Magnetic resonance imaging with its ability to visualize sagittal sections of the body is very successful at demonstrating lesions within the spinal cord and it has rapidly become the investigation of choice in this condition.

Treatment

Treatment is surgical and depends on decompressing the craniovertebral junction in an attempt to normalize the flow of CSF. A ventriculoperitoneal shunt is sometimes inserted to prevent raised pressure within the ventricular system being transmitted to the syrinx. Unfortunately, it is rare for these procedures to be followed by much clinical improvement; the most that can be hoped is that the progression of the condition will be arrested.

TRANSVERSE MYELITIS

Transverse myelitis is an inflammatory condition involving both grey and white matter of the spinal cord. It may occur at any level of the cord but is most common in the thoracic region. The longitudinal extent of the lesion is confined to a few segments. Transverse myelitis may occur as a complication of several diseases:

1. Multiple sclerosis
2. Viral infection
   a. Coxsackie viruses
   b. Other enteroviruses
   c. Herpes zoster
   d. Epstein-Barr virus
3. Postinfectious
   a. Chickenpox
   b. Measles
   c. Postvaccination against smallpox
4. Systemic lupus erythematosus.

Clinical features

Onset is dramatic with a flaccid paraplegia developing over a period of a few hours to a few days. Bladder control is almost always affected. Sensory changes affecting all modalities develop below the level of the lesion. There is often a clearly delineated sensory level sometimes with a zone of hyperaesthesia just above the level of reduced or absent sensation. The patient is often pyrexial and may complain of back pain.

Investigations

Except in cases where the clinical diagnosis is quite clear, myelography is necessary in order to exclude a compressive lesion of the spinal cord.

The CSF shows a raised protein content and a mononuclear pleocytosis. Serological and CSF antibody studies may allow a specific diagnosis when the cause is viral.

Prognosis and treatment

Considering the severity of the clinical features in the acute stages, the prognosis for recovery is surprisingly good. Treatment follows the principles for care of the paraplegic patient. There is some evidence that ACTH or steroids may be of value.

INFARCTION OF THE SPINAL CORD

On the dorsal surface the two posterior spinal arteries form an anastomotic network and the dorsal third of the spinal cord, which these arteries supply, is relatively protected against occlusion of a single vessel. By contrast, the single anterior spinal artery, which runs longitudinally down the ventral surface of the cord and supplies the ventral two-thirds, is fed from only a few vessels. The cervical segment of the artery is fed from the vertebral arteries; the thoracic segment by a few vessels derived directly from the aorta, usually at about the level of T10. Occlusion of one of these thoracic branches as a result of embolism or thrombosis, or as a complication of cervical or thoracic surgery is likely to produce an ischaemic zone in the watershed upper thoracic region and result in acute paraparesis.

There is sudden onset of weakness of both legs with signs of bilateral corticospinal tract lesions. Pain and temperature sensation are lost, but vibration and joint position sensation are preserved. Control of sphincter is affected. In the acute stages there is often severe interscapular pain. Some degree of recovery is possible, particularly when the lesion is incomplete.

CARE OF THE PARAPLEGIC PATIENT

The first step in the management of a paraplegic patient is to establish the cause of the paraplegia. Some of the causes and their investigation and treatment have been discussed earlier in this chapter. Whether or not specific treatment is available, great care and attention will be necessary to avoid the complications of the paraplegia itself.

Bladder problems

Catheterization to prevent urinary retention and consequent distension of the bladder is required from the time of onset of the paraplegia. Regular intermittent catheterization may be preferable to leaving a catheter in place because it increases the chances of the patient eventually developing reflex autonomic bladder function. Urinary tract infection is a constant hazard and prompt treatment with antibiotics when an infection develops is necessary.

Skin care

A paraplegic patient is very likely to develop pressure sores because of his sensory loss. Nursing patients on an air-bed lessens the risk, but strict attention to regular and frequent turning will still be necessary.

Contractures

Intensive physiotherapy beginning as soon as possible after the onset of the paraplegia is essential to prevent the development of contractures and tendon shortening.

Rehabilitation

Referral of the patient to a spinal injuries centre after the acute stage of the illness is past provides the best chance of minimizing his long-term disability. Treatment will depend on how much independent function remains. Techniques such as tendon transplants in which the tendon of a functioning muscle is reimplanted to give a more useful movement may have a place in helping the patient to be as independent as possible in the activities of daily life. Expert advice concerning adaption of the patient's home and place of work as well as the most useful aids is required.

25. Low back pain

Low back pain is a very common complaint and probably affects the majority of people at some time in their lives. Many of the causes are mechanical and related to degenerative disease of the intervertebral discs or the posterior intervertebral joints. Other causes of back pain include osteoporosis, Paget's disease, inflammatory conditions such as ankylosing spondylitis and bony metastatic deposits from primary neoplasms of lung, breast, kidney and prostate. Most patients with these conditions never develop neurological complications and are looked after by rheumatologists, general physicians or orthopaedic surgeons. A small proportion, however, present to a neurologist because of symptoms of nerve root irritation or compression of the cauda equina.

LUMBAR DISC PROLAPSE

Mechanism

The intervertebral discs that form the flexible fibrous joints between vertebral bodies consist of a tough outer ring, the annulus, surrounding a soft central core, the nucleus pulposus. Degeneration of the disc with age or as a result of repeated minor trauma allows herniation of the nucleus through a defect in the annulus. The precipitating event is often comparatively minor; disc prolapse may occur when getting out of a car or standing up from a stooping position. Most disc prolapses point laterally within the spinal canal where their position allows them to impinge on an adjacent nerve root and cause pain in the distribution of that root. Central disc prolapse also occurs and this may result in compression of the cauda equina.

The vast majority of disc prolapses occur at the L4/5 or L5/S1 levels. Because of the anatomical arrangement of the lumbar and sacral nerve roots, a lateral disc prolapse usually affects the root immediately below the level of prolapse. A disc prolapse at the L4/5 level therefore tends to cause symptoms referable to the L5 root and a prolapse at L5/S1 level to cause symptoms in the S1 root.

Clinical features of lumbar nerve root compression

The patient can often describe the event which preceded the symptoms. There is severe pain in the distribution of the affected nerve root and dull aching in the lower part of the back. Root pain is exacerbated by coughing or straining. Paraesthesia and numbness may be present in the area innervated by the affected root.

When examined, the patient shows restriction of passive straight-leg raising. Normally, with the patient lying flat, the leg can be raised to an angle of 80°−90° from the horizontal. In cases where a lateral disc prolapse abuts a nerve root, the pain caused by increased tension on the root as the leg is raised may prevent the leg being lifted beyond about 45°. If, while the leg is raised, the examiner increases tension on the nerve root by pressing on the tibial nerve in the popliteal fossa or dorsiflexing the foot, pain is exacerbated (Fig. 25.1). Flexing the knee decreases tension on the root and relieves the pain. Weakness in muscles innervated by the affected root may be present and there may also be sensory changes in the corresponding dermatome. If the S1 root is affected the ankle jerk is often depressed.

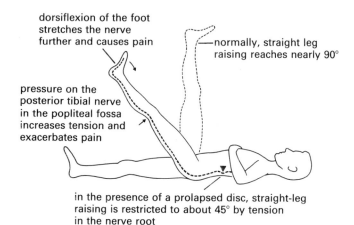

dorsiflexion of the foot stretches the nerve further and causes pain

normally, straight leg raising reaches nearly 90°

pressure on the posterior tibial nerve in the popliteal fossa increases tension and exacerbates pain

in the presence of a prolapsed disc, straight-leg raising is restricted to about 45° by tension in the nerve root

Fig. 25.1 Straight-leg raising.

Treatment

In most patients with root irritation from acute disc prolapse, symptoms settle after one or two weeks' bed rest. It is usual to advise placing a board under the mattress. After the acute symptoms have settled, a course of physiotherapy to strengthen the extensors of the spine may speed up the process of remobilization.

Epidural injections of local anaesthetic are often effective in relieving the acute symptoms of lumbar disc prolapse but, in practice, it may be difficult to arrange for the injection to be given quickly enough to be of much benefit.

Patients who have recovered from disc prolapse should be advised to avoid heavy lifting and instructed how to reach objects on the ground by squatting down rather than bending over.

Recurrent attacks of back pain and sciatica, or symptoms which fail to settle after a prolonged period of rest are the main indications for further investigation and surgical intervention. Radiculography is necessary to confirm that the symptoms are caused by prolapse of an intervertebral disc and to establish at which level the prolapse has occurred. The usual surgical approach is to perform a laminectomy and to decompress the affected nerve root.

Central disc prolapse

Prolapse of a lumbar disc centrally is much less common but potentially far more serious than a lateral disc prolapse because multiple nerve roots of the cauda equina are at risk of compression. Symptoms and signs vary according to the level and extent of the prolapse, but the usual presentation is pain in the back which radiates down both legs, weakness in both legs usually most marked in muscles innervated by L5 and S1 roots (dorsiflexors and plantarflexors of the foot) and retention of urine. Sensory loss over the lower sacral dermatomes (saddle area) is present.

Immediate investigation by myelography is required. Unless surgical decompression is undertaken urgently the chances of functional recovery of bladder function are small.

OTHER CAUSES OF LUMBAR AND SACRAL NERVE ROOT LESIONS

A number of spinal tumours including neurofibromas, ependymomas, lipomas and dermoid cysts arise in the lumbar and sacral regions of the spinal canal. Root pain which fails to settle with bed rest or pain that affects roots other than L5 or S1 should raise the suspicion that the cause is something other than a prolapse of an intervertebral disc. Early myelography to investigate the nature of the lesion is indicated in these circumstances.

LUMBAR SPINAL CANAL STENOSIS

There is considerable individual variation in the internal dimensions of the spinal canal. In people with a congenitally narrow canal, degenerative disease may reduce the diameter further and cause a chronic syndrome of nerve root compression. The bulging annulus fibrosus of the degenerating intervertebral disc and associated osteophyte formation at the posterior margins of the vertebral bodies narrow the canal anteriorly. Thickening of the ligamentum flavum and degenerative changes around the posterior intervertebral joints narrow the canal posteriorly. A history of trauma to the lumbar spine is commonly obtained.

Clinical features

The characteristic clinical picture is of root pain, which may be bilateral, brought on by exercise and relieved by rest. The features may easily be confused with intermittent claudication caused by occlusive disease of peripheral arteries. Distinguishing features are the root distribution of the pain in spinal stenosis compared with the calf pain of vascular claudication and the development of clinical signs of sensory or motor disturbance following exercise.

Treatment

Myelography or CT scanning of the lumbar spine after the injection of intrathecal contrast medium demonstrates narrowing of the spinal canal and compression of the nerve roots of the cauda equina. Surgical treatment by extensive laminectomy is usually effective.

26. Motor neurone disease

Motor neurone disease is an uncommon condition with an incidence of 1–2 per 100 000 population per year. It rarely occurs before the age of 50 years, but the incidence increases with age. The cause is quite unknown despite intensive efforts to follow up what seemed an important epidemiological clue—the very high incidence of the disease on the island of Guam in the Western Pacific.

The pathological features of the disease are loss of lower motor neurones from the anterior horn of spinal cord grey matter and the motor nuclei of the lower cranial nerves, loss of nerve cells from the motor cortex of the cerebral hemispheres and degeneration of the corticospinal tracts in the spinal cord.

Subdivisions of the disease into amyotrophic lateral sclerosis, progressive bulbar palsy and progressive muscular atrophy are sometimes made. These distinctions depend on the clinical manifestations; whether it is limb or bulbar muscles that are mainly affected and whether the disease predominantly involves lower or upper motor neurones. In most patients the disease will eventually progress to involve both upper and lower motor neurones and both bulbar and limb muscles, regardless of the symptoms at presentation, and differentiation between the different forms is no longer thought very helpful.

Clinical features

The commonest presentation is with fatigue and weakness in one limb. Less often the bulbar muscles are affected first and the patient presents with dysphagia and dysarthria. Painful muscle cramps may be a feature. Although the signs and symptoms may be confined to one group of muscles at presentation, the disease is inexorably progressive leading to death within a few years. The terminal event is often aspiration pneumonia.

Examination reveals both upper and lower motor neurone signs. Brisk tendon jerks and extensor plantar responses point to the involvement of upper motor neurones. Evidence of disease of lower motor neurones is seen in the wasted and fasciculating muscles. This combination of pathologically brisk tendon reflexes and wasted muscles is characteristic of motor neurone disease.

When the lower cranial nerves are affected there are features of a pseudobulbar palsy—spastic dysarthria, palatal weakness, difficulty in initiating swallowing, a brisk jaw jerk and emotional lability—with additional signs of lower motor neurone loss, usually seen most clearly in the fasciculating tongue. Despite the severity of the involvement of the lower cranial nerves the oculomotor nerves are almost never affected. Sphincter control remains intact and clinical examination of sensation is normal.

Treatment

No treatment is known which alters the relentless course of the disease. Some publicity has recently been given to assertions that intravenous injections of TRH in massive doses result in improved muscle strength. Evaluated in controlled conditions, these claims were less impressive and, in any case, the very short-lived improvement offered little hope for a useful treatment.

Symptomatic and palliative measures should not be neglected. Cricopharyngeal myotomy is a useful procedure to alleviate dysphagia in cases where features of a pseudobulbar palsy predominate. A fine-bore nasogastric tube or a feeding gastrostomy may also be helpful. When dysarthria and dysphonia are severe enough to prevent useful speech an electronic communication aid should be provided. As muscle strength deteriorates walking aids and wheelchairs may be needed. Patients with motor neurone disease need to be assessed by someone with experience of the disease and with knowledge of the aids available. The progressive nature of the disease means that a patient will become increasingly disabled. It is therefore essential that the aids are supplied promptly and their usefulness frequently reviewed.

27. Cerebellar disorders

A cerebellar syndrome of ataxia, dysarthria and nystagmus may result from a variety of lesions of both the cerebellum and its connections. Lesions affecting the midline structures of the cerebellum, the vermis and the flocculo-nodular lobe, cause ataxia of gait and disturbance of balance. When disease affects the cerebellar hemispheres ataxia of limbs tends to predominate.

Space-occupying lesions of the cerebellum and posterior fossa often cause an obstructive hydrocephalus and symptoms of raised intracranial pressure because of the close anatomical relation to the 4th ventricle and the foramina through which CSF exits from the ventricular system of the brain.

Cerebellar dysfunction may also be part of the clinical picture of more widespread disease in the nervous system, such as in multiple sclerosis or cerebrovascular disease. The cerebellum is also a common site for metastatic tumour deposits.

The age of the patient is one of the most important ways of narrowing down the differential diagnosis.

DISORDERS OF ONSET IN CHILDHOOD

Friedreich's ataxia

This is a familial disorder, usually inherited as an autosomal recessive trait, which first presents in childhood or adolescence. The pathological features of the disease are degeneration of the dorsal columns, the corticospinal tracts and the spinocerebellar tracts of the spinal cord. The lower part of the cord is more severely affected than the cervical segments, which explains why the earliest clinical features are usually ataxia of gait and spasticity of the lower limbs. The disease is progressive, gradually involving the upper limbs and causing dysarthria, irregular head movements and nystagmus. Optic atrophy and pes cavus are present in the majority of cases.

Acute cerebellar ataxia of infancy

A syndrome of acute cerebellar ataxia in very young children sometimes follows chickenpox, one of the other acute exanthemata of childhood or a non-specific infection. Although the ataxia may be so severe that the child is unable even to sit without support, the prognosis is good and full recovery within a few weeks or months is usual. The pathogenesis is probably autoimmune of a similar type to that found in postinfectious encephalomyelitis.

Cerebellar tumours

Medulloblastoma is a midline tumour arising in the roof of the 4th ventricle. It usually occurs in children under the age of 10 years and, because of its position, causes an obstructive hydrocephalus and raised intracranial pressure at an early stage. It is radiosensitive and surgical removal followed by radiotherapy is successful in a high proportion of cases.

Astrocytomas of the cerebellar hemisphere are less common but they, too, nearly always occur in childhood. They present with features of ataxia, often confined to the ipsilateral hand, nystagmus and hypotonia. The symptoms are frequently remarkably slight when compared with the size of the tumour.

DISORDERS OF ONSET IN ADULT LIFE

Progressive cerebellar degeneration

This term is used to describe a group of degenerative conditions beginning in middle age. The clinical features include limb and gait ataxia, dysarthria and, more variably, tremor, spasticity, extrapyramidal features and mental deterioration. A number of varieties of cerebellar degeneration have been described: primary parenchymatous degeneration of the cerebellum, delayed cortical cerebellar atrophy, olivopontocerebellar atrophy, Sanger Brown's spinocerebellar ataxia and Marie's spastic ataxia. Whether these are truly distinct entities is uncertain. In some cases the condition is familial.

Metabolic and toxic causes

Hypothyroidism, long-term treatment with anticonvulsants, especially phenytoin, and chronic alcohol abuse have all been occasionally associated with cerebellar degeneration. Degeneration
of the cerebellum is also sometimes seen as a non-metastatic complication of carcinoma of the lung.

Cerebellar tumours

Primary cerebellar tumours are rare in adults. In contrast, the
cerebellum is a common site for metastatic tumour from lung and
breast and from cutaneous melanoma.

28. Facial palsy and facial pain

All the muscles of facial expression, including those which close the eye, are innervated by the facial nerve. The part of the facial nerve nucleus that sends lower motor neurones to orbicularis oculi and frontalis receives a bilateral upper motor neurone innervation from the motor cortex. Unilateral upper motor neurone lesions of facial innervation therefore spare the upper part of the face. In contrast, lower motor neurone lesions, situated either in the nucleus itself or in the peripheral part of the facial nerve, cause weakness that affects the whole of the ipsilateral side of the face. For a more detailed account of the neuroanatomy of the facial nerve see Chapter 4.

The sensory nerve supply to the face is by the trigeminal nerve. The anatomy of this nerve is also described in Chapter 4.

SUPRANUCLEAR (UPPER MOTOR NEURONE) FACIAL WEAKNESS

The presence of unilateral weakness of the lower part of the face, while the ability to close the eye and wrinkle the skin of the forehead remain intact, indicates a contralateral supranuclear lesion of facial innervation. This pattern is commonly seen in the victims of stroke where, in addition to a hemiplegia, the lower part of one side of the face is also weak. Other causes of supranuclear facial weakness include multiple sclerosis and neoplasms.

LOWER MOTOR NEURONE CAUSES OF FACIAL WEAKNESS

Bell's palsy

The eponym refers to a disorder of unknown aetiology in which swelling and inflammation of the facial nerve within the facial canal results in unilateral facial weakness. Bell's palsy is the commonest cause of facial palsy of the lower motor neurone type.

Clinical features

The development of unilateral facial weakness is frequently preceded by pain behind the ear. This may last a day or two and can be quite severe. Apart from the facial weakness the patient may complain of hyperacusis (because the branch of the facial nerve which innervates stapedius is affected); reduced salivation (because the greater superficial petrosal nerve which carries secretomotor fibres to the sublingual and submandibular salivary glands is part of the facial nerve); and impaired taste on one side of the tongue (because sensory nerve fibres carrying taste sensation from the anterior two-thirds of the tongue travel with the facial nerve in the facial canal).

Examination

The appearance of the face is obviously asymmetrical. Asking the patient to show his teeth reveals that movement of one side of the mouth is diminished or absent. When the patient tries to close his eye he exhibits Bell's phenomenon—the eyeball rotates upward but the eyelid fails to descend. Lacrimation is rarely affected in cases of Bell's palsy, but the patient may complain of a weepy eye because the loss of tone in the lower eyelid tends to allow tears to roll down his cheek instead of draining into the nasolacrimal duct.

Treatment

Treatment with high doses of steroids is often given for a short period in the belief that inflammation and oedema of the facial nerve will be reduced. There is no good evidence from controlled trials that this treatment is of benefit. The majority of patients, especially if they are young or the facial palsy is incomplete, make a full recovery in 2−3 months. In the remainder some degree of facial weakness persists indefinitely.

Geniculate herpes zoster

Herpes zoster infection of the facial (geniculate) ganglion causes a painful vesicular eruption within the external auditory meatus

Table 28.1 Other causes of unilateral facial palsy

Site of lesion in the facial nerve	Pathology
Within the brain stem	Vascular lesions Demyelination
In the cerebellopontine angle	Acoustic neuroma
Within the subarachnoid space	Leukaemic or carcinomatous deposits
Within the facial canal	Basal skull fracture Middle ear infection
Distal to the stylomastoid foramen	Parotid gland tumours Sarcoidosis

and over the anterior pillar of the fauces. A lower motor neurone type of facial palsy and loss of taste over one side of the tongue occur in association. This condition is sometimes known as the Ramsay Hunt syndrome, but beware of this designation because the same eponym is also given to a very rare degenerative disease of the cerebellum.

Other causes of facial palsy are summarized in Table 28.1.

Bilateral facial weakness

Bilateral facial weakness is harder to recognize at a glance than unilateral weakness because symmetry of the face is maintained. A routine of testing the power of the facial muscles by asking the patient to smile, to puff out his cheeks and to screw up his eyes ensures that the condition is not overlooked. It is important to remember that bilateral weakness of the face may be caused by disease of muscle or the neuromuscular junction as well as by bilateral lesions of the facial nerve.

Causes of bilateral facial weakness are:

1. Bell's palsy is bilateral on rare occasions
2. Sarcoidosis
3. Lyme disease
4. Myasthenia gravis
5. Dystrophia myotonica
6. Facioscapulohumeral muscular dystrophy
7. Intrinsic lesions of the pons.

Hemifacial spasm

This peculiar condition usually affects middle-aged women. In the early stages there are frequent but intermittent attacks of fine rapid twitching in the lateral part of orbicularis oculi. Over a long period the spasms spread to involve the muscles of the lower part of the face. Eventually weakness or even complete paralysis of the affected side develops.

Some believe that the condition is caused by irritation of the facial nerve by a tortuosity in a nearby blood vessel and there are reports that surgical intervention, in which the nerve is dissected free of blood vessels, produces good results. No drug treatment is of lasting benefit.

Trigeminal neuralgia

Trigeminal neuralgia mainly affects people over the age of 50 years and women more frequently than men. There is usually no identifiable cause, but it may rarely be a symptom of multiple sclerosis (this diagnosis should be suspected if the patient is young) or of a tumour in the cerebellopontine angle.

Clinical features

The patient experiences sudden attacks of intense pain within the distribution of one of the divisions of the trigeminal nerve. Most commonly the pain radiates from around the mouth towards the ear, or from the upper lip into the nostril and the lower eyelid. Trigeminal neuralgia very rarely affects the ophthalmic division of the nerve. Patients describe the pain as shooting or stabbing and leave no doubt about its severity. Each paroxysm of pain lasts only a short time, but if the attacks are recurring frequently there may be a background of pain between the attacks. Pain is often precipitated by jaw movement or by touching the face in a particular spot. Simple actions like chewing, speaking, washing the face or brushing the teeth can trigger an attack.

Examination

If trigeminal neuralgia is a symptom of a tumour, examination will reveal sensory loss in the distribution of the trigeminal nerve and probably other signs suggesting a cerebellopontine angle lesion (see p. 192). In the idiopathic form of the condition there are no physical signs. Unfortunately, this distinction may not be so easy to make in practice as it is in theory. Patients with trigeminal neuralgia are reluctant to allow the lightest touch in the affected area out of fear that an attack of pain will be precipitated.

Treatment

Treatment with carbamazepine almost always improves symptoms and may abolish them altogether. Baclofen and phenytoin may also be effective. For those patients who respond poorly to drug treatment there are a variety of surgical procedures, including section of the affected division of the nerve, injection of alcohol or phenol into the trigeminal ganglion and radiofrequency thermocoagulation of the ganglion. They all carry the disadvantage of producing a degree of facial anaesthesia, which, if it involves the cornea, is a serious problem.

Trigeminal neuropathy

Trigeminal neuropathy is an uncommon condition, sometimes associated with connective tissue disease, particularly systemic sclerosis, in which there is slowly progressive bilateral sensory loss of the central part of the face. Investigations usually fail to reveal any underlying cause and the pathogenesis remains a mystery.

Postherpetic neuralgia

Following ophthalmic Herpes zoster some patients continue to suffer severe pain despite resolution of the vesicular eruption. The pain is burning in character and continuous but stimulation of the skin over the affected area may exacerbate the pain. In a few cases symptoms improve with time but in most the pain persists indefinitely. Response to treatment is very variable; some patients derive great benefit from transcutaneous nerve stimulation or from tricyclic antidepressants, but in others the pain is intractable. Unlike trigeminal neuralgia, postherpetic neuralgia rarely responds to carbamazepine.

Atypical facial pain

This is a rather unsatisfactorily defined condition, almost exclusively confined to middle-aged women who complain of an aching, boring pain in the lower part of the face usually over the cheek. Investigations show no neurological, dental or sinus disease and it is often thought that the problem is psychogenic. This conclusion tends to be reinforced by the apparently exaggerated descriptions of the severity of the pain which are often given by the patient.

Treatment with tricyclic antidepressants is often effective, even in the absence of any overt features of depression.

Other causes of facial pain

A variety of non-neurological conditions also produce facial pain. Arthritis of the temporomandibular joint resulting from dental malocclusion causes pain over the side of the face that is exacerbated by chewing and other movements of the jaw. Other causes of pain in the face include disease of the teeth and infection of the paranasal air sinuses.

29. Headache

INTRODUCTION

Headache is a common reason for referral to a neurological out-patient clinic. Although an organic reason for the headache will be found in only a very small proportion of patients, there are at least three good reasons for taking a careful history and perform-ing a full examination in every patient. First, it will prevent any serious organic cause for the headache being overlooked; second, many patients with functional headache respond well to ap-propriate treatment and third, the fact that a patient has attended a clinic is a tacit sign that he has become worried either about the cause of the headache or about the effect it is having on his life. Only if the doctor's approach demonstrates that he is taking the patient's complaint seriously will reassurance about the benign nature of the symptoms carry any weight.

No classification has been completely successful in integrating the causes, symptoms and pathophysiology of headache. This is partly because of the large number of varieties of headache that have been described whose cause and mechanism can only be speculated about and partly because headache seems a uniquely human complaint whose pathological mechanisms cannot be in-vestigated in animals. The headings used in this chapter are based on cause where the condition is organic and symptoms where the condition is functional.

ORGANIC CAUSES OF HEADACHE

Intracranial space-occupying lesions

Intracranial space-occupying lesions, whether neoplasm, abscess or haematoma, cause headache if they exert traction on or distort the dura or intracranial blood vessels, these structures being pain sensitive. They can also cause headache by interfering with the normal circulation of CSF to produce raised intracranial pressure. The headache of raised intracranial pressure is felt as a dull pain over the whole of the head, worst on waking in the morning and exacerbated by coughing, straining and bending. In advanced cases the headache is associated with sudden vomiting, often in the absence of a preceding feeling of nausea, and transient obscuration of vision. Examination is likely to reveal papilloedema and focal neurological signs related to the site of the lesion. Urgent investigation by CT scanning is required.

Meningeal irritation

Irritation of the meninges by acute infection or the presence of blood in the subarachnoid space causes severe headache. The headache is accompanied by signs of meningeal irritation—neck stiffness and a positive Kernig's sign (see Fig. 9.1). That the headache is a symptom of organic disease is usually obvious from the patient's general condition and there is very rarely any difficulty in diagnosing the underlying cause. The clinical features of bacterial and viral meningitis and subarachnoid haemorrhage are described on pages 177 and 159 respectively.

Giant cell arteritis

Giant cell arteritis is an uncommon condition, rarely occurring before the age of 50 and more frequent in women than men. Autopsies carried out on cases who died in the acute phase of the disease have shown an inflammatory process in the walls of the superficial temporal, vertebral, ophthalmic and posterior ciliary arteries, which indicates that the disease is more widespread than the alternative name *temporal arteritis* suggests. The inflammatory process involves all layers of the arterial wall with thickening, round cell infiltration and giant cell formation. Sites of inflammation are distributed patchily along the artery—so called skip lesions.

Clinical features

Constant unilateral or bilateral headache with tenderness over the distribution of the temporal artery is the major symptom. In addition, there may be general malaise, aching and stiffness in neck and shoulder muscles and pain on chewing. This last symptom is sometimes called jaw claudication. Physicians with a taste for the flashy sometimes claim to be able to make an instant diagnosis of giant cell arteritis if a well-dressed elderly woman walks into their consulting rooms with unbrushed hair; the deranged hairstyle is the clue that points to the scalp tenderness.

Examination reveals a thickened, tender, non-pulsating superficial temporal artery. The ESR is usually very high. A temporal artery biopsy should be carried out in an attempt to confirm the diagnosis but, because of the patchy distribution of the lesions, false negative biopsies are not unusual. A negative biopsy from a patient with a good history of giant cell arteritis, especially if the ESR is raised, should not prevent treatment with steroids.

Treatment

Giant cell arteritis is a medical emergency because, untreated, there is a very significant risk of blindness from thrombosis of the ophthalmic or posterior ciliary arteries. Treatment should be started with 60 mg of prednisolone daily without waiting for the results of the biopsy. After a few weeks the dose can be gradually reduced using the ESR to monitor the effectiveness of treatment. Steroids must usually be continued for 12 months or more.

Disease of paranasal sinuses and bones of the skull

Infection of the paranasal air sinuses is very common and often painful. The pain tends to be localized to the infected sinus and pressure over the affected sinus increases the pain. A rare complication, if the ostium of the sinus becomes completely blocked, is the development of a mucocele. It may slowly enlarge, eroding bone and expanding into the orbit or the anterior cranial fossa.

Paget's disease affects the skull quite commonly. The most important neurological complication is the development of cranial nerve palsies as a result of narrowing of the exit foramina of the nerves by the overgrowth of bone but sometimes the hyperaemic bone is painful and patients with Paget's disease of the skull occasionally present with a complaint of headache.

FUNCTIONAL CAUSES OF HEADACHE

Migraine

Migraine is the name given to recurrent headaches, often affecting only one side of the head, sometimes throbbing in character, usually accompanied by nausea and photophobia and sometimes by vomiting too. The headaches may be preceded by visual or sensory symptoms, known as a migrainous aura, and also by changes in mood. Different varieties of migraine are recognized and not all these features need be present in an individual patient in order to make the diagnosis.

The pathophysiology of migraine is only poorly understood. Most attention has been focused on the classical type of migraine in which the headache is preceded by a brief period of neurological disturbance. Measurement of regional cerebral blood flow during the aura of classical migraine has demonstrated both general and focal reductions of perfusion followed, during the headache phase of the attack, by an increased blood flow in intracranial and extracranial circulations. It is not known whether the depression in cortical activity that causes the symptoms of the aura of classical migraine is a result of ischaemia or whether the reduction in blood flow is itself secondary to the diminished cortical activity.

Parallels have been drawn between the migrainous aura and the phenomenon of spreading cortical depression that has been observed in the brains of experimental animals. In reaction to local trauma, dehydration or hypoxia waves of inhibition spread across the cerebral cortex at a rate of a few millimetres per second and suppress normal cortical activity. Spreading depression is associated with an initial vasoconstriction and subsequent vasodilatation and it has been argued that this indicates that the primary event in migraine takes place in the cortex and not in the cerebral blood vessels.

The mechanism of the production of pain during the headache phase of an attack of migraine is also the subject of controversy. Dilatation of extracranial and meningeal blood vessels, whose walls have been rendered hypersensitive to distension by release of 5-hydroxytryptamine from platelets, has been suggested as an explanation.

Classical migraine

This type of migraine is characterized by a prodromal neurological disturbance. Commonly, this originates in the visual cortex of the occipital lobe. Primitive visual hallucinations of white or coloured zig-zags, sometimes known as *fortification spectra* or *teichopsia*, expand across the visual field leaving a scotoma of impaired vision behind them. Other visual manifestations of migraine are sudden flashes of light, usually in the peripheral part of the visual field, a shimmering central scotoma or a homonymous hemianopia. Less frequently, there may be a unilateral sensory or motor disturbance—paraesthesia in an arm or leg, or a feeling of heaviness down one side of the body. Rarely, if the temporal or parietal lobes are involved, more complex feelings of altered perception occur.

The neurological disturbance usually, but not always, precedes the headache. It is rare for it to persist for longer than 30 minutes. The accompanying headache is usually severe and associated with strong feelings of nausea and repeated vomiting. The sufferer is photophobic and wants nothing else but to lie down in a quiet and darkened room.

Migraine equivalents

Occasionally, a sufferer from classical migraine experiences the prodromal features of migraine without any following headache, nausea or vomiting. These phenomena are known as migraine equivalents.

Common migraine

Unilateral throbbing headaches associated with nausea, vomiting, anorexia and photophobia, but without prodromal neurological features are termed common migraine. Many patients suffer from headaches with some but not all of these features and it may be difficult to decide whether their symptoms really amount to migraine or whether they would be more accurately labelled as having tension headache.

Basilar artery migraine

In this rare variety of migraine, which mainly affects young women, the migrainous aura consists of symptoms of brain stem disturbance such as diplopia, dysarthria, vertigo, ataxia and loss of consciousness. The accompanying headache is predominantly occipital.

Ophthalmoplegic migraine

A rare sequel to an attack of migraine is transient diplopia caused by a 3rd or 6th nerve palsy. Unlike other neurological disturbances in migraine the ophthalmoplegia follows the headache instead of preceding it. The probable explanation is that dilatation of the internal carotid artery within the cavernous sinus has compressed one of the oculomotor nerves. The condition usually recovers completely in a few days. Because headache and ophthalmoplegia can also be symptoms of expanding aneurysms of the posterior part of the circle of Willis, investigation is necessary.

Complicated migraine

Migraine is, for the vast majority of sufferers, an unpleasant but benign condition. Very occasionally, the neurological disturbance of the migrainous aura may persist for several days or even become permanent. The mechanism may be that the phase of vasoconstriction was so intense that infarction of cerebral cortex resulted, or that thrombotic occlusion of an artery occurred as a result of the reduction in blood flow. Hemiplegia or visual field defects are the commonest complications of migraine. Hemiplegic migraine is sometimes familial.

Treatment of migraine

The acute attack is best treated with simple analgesics and antiemetics. Ergotamine, taken as early as possible during the attack, is effective in some patients with classical migraine. Unfortunately, it often causes vomiting. The drug has a powerful and prolonged vasoconstrictor action and patients must be warned not to take more than a total of 3 mg in a week. Some sufferers from migraine find that if they can lie down in a darkened room they can abort the attack by going to sleep.

If severe attacks of migraine are occurring more often than about once a fortnight, or are seriously interfering with a patient's life or work, prophylactic medication should be considered. Propranolol, pizotifen and methysergide are all moderately effective in the prophylaxis of migraine. Propranolol given in a dose of 40–80 mg three times daily has been shown to be effective in double-blind trials and is free of serious adverse effects providing patients with a history of asthma are excluded. Pizotifen has also clearly been shown to be effective, but it has the disadvantage of being sedating and, in women particularly, of causing a craving for sweet foods. Patients must be warned of this so that they can avoid gaining weight. Methysergide carries a risk of causing retroperitoneal fibrosis; the risk is very small but because the consequences are so serious the drug should be avoided as far as possible. It is thought that the risk of retroperitoneal fibrosis is reduced if the drug is withdrawn for one month in six.

Some patients with migraine are able to identify factors which precipitate attacks. These may be dietary, related to menstruation or linked to emotional states. It is worth exploring the possibility that minor modifications in the way a patient organizes his life might reduce the frequency of migraine.

Tension headache

Tension headache is the commonest of all the varieties of headache. Indeed, patients sometimes describe it as a 'normal' headache and many, if not most, of the readers of this book will have experienced it at sometime in their lives. It is felt as a dull ache or pressure on the top of the head or as a constricting band in the frontal or temporal regions. It is absent on waking and comes on gradually during the course of the day. Rarely does it interfere with sleep. Sometimes there are local points of tenderness on the scalp over frontalis, occipitalis or temporalis muscles.

The clinical characteristics of tension headache and common migraine form a continuous spectrum. Many patients with some features of tension headache describe symptoms of vague nausea or a throbbing component to their headache and, as mentioned previously, it may be impossible to categorize their headache definitely as tension headache or common migraine. The terms combined headache or tension-vascular headache are sometimes used for these cases.

One theory of tension headache is that it arises from pain in the muscles of the scalp caused by excessive contraction. It is certainly true that gritting of the teeth and furrowing of the brow are ways in which irritation, anxiety and stress may be manifested. Unfortunately, electromyographic studies of the activity of these muscles in patients with tension headache have given equivocal results and the theory is far from proven.

Treatment

Tension headache becomes a medical problem when the symptoms are chronic. A proportion of patients with chronic tension headache are aware that their symptoms are related to stress, either at home or at work, and only want reassurance that their headaches are not caused by any serious neurological disease. In others it is impossible to uncover any underlying psychological reason for their symptoms. Most patients have already tried treating themselves with simple analgesics and have found them of little help. Tricyclic antidepressants in low dose are sometimes very effective in treating tension headache, even when there are no indications of a depressive illness. Benzodiazepines should be avoided.

Cluster headache

Cluster headache is an unusual condition almost exclusively affecting men. It has several alternative names, including *migrainous neuralgia, histamine cephalgia* and *Horton's cephalgia*. They all refer to a syndrome of short-lived, but severe, unilateral headache localized around the orbit. Reddening and suffusion of the conjunctiva, lacrimation and rhinorrhoea usually accompany the orbital pain. Sometimes a Horner's syndrome develops transiently in association. Each attack lasts between 60 and 90 minutes but the patient may suffer several attacks each day. Frequently the attack wakes the patient from sleep in the early hours of the morning. The pain may be very severe; patients describe walking around the house desperately trying to think of some way of obtaining relief. They often volunteer that, when the attack is at its height, they feel like banging their head against a wall. This pattern of behaviour is quite unlike that of someone suffering an attack of migraine. Most patients with migraine only want to remain quietly in a darkened room until the attack subsides.

The name cluster headache derives from the peculiar way in which the attacks are clustered together in time. A patient may have several attacks each day for a month or six weeks and then be entirely free of headache for many months. A peculiar feature of cluster headache is that, during a cluster, the headaches always recur on the same side.

Treatment

Because each attack is so short-lived it is often not practical to try to treat the attack when it occurs. The aim should be prophylaxis. Ergotamine taken at night before the patient goes to bed is often effective in preventing nocturnal attacks, but the treatment cannot be continued for more than a week or two because of the danger of causing peripheral ischaemia. Short courses of corticosteroids, pizotifen and lithium carbonate are also of value in some patients.

30. Dementia

The term dementia refers to a generalized deterioration of higher mental functions in a patient whose level of consciousness is unimpaired. The earliest features of dementia are failure of memory, a decline in the ability to make reasoned judgements, loss of the correct use of social skills and loss of control of emotional reactions. The patient usually has little insight into his condition but sometimes, in the first stages of the illness, he may be aware that tasks which he could previously undertake without difficulty are now beyond him. This often leads to changes in mood, usually towards depression, and disturbances of behaviour as the patient tries to express his frustration and bewilderment. As the dementia becomes more severe, patients begin to neglect their appearance and fail to attend to matters of personal hygiene. Dysphasic speech difficulties, apraxia and incontinence are later features. In the last stages of dementia patients require constant care by others; they are unable to communicate, to wash and dress, or even to feed themselves.

Dementia is a syndrome rather than a specific disease. There are a large number of possible causes (Table 30.1) but, unfortunately, most of them are progressive and resistant to treatment. The two commonest causes, Alzheimer's disease and multiple cerebral infarction, are much more frequent in the elderly. The ageing population of most countries in the Western world means that the prevalence of dementia is increasing rapidly. The high degree of care that these patients demand places a heavy burden on their relatives and on medical resources.

When dealing with a patient who presents with intellectual impairment, deterioration in memory, or other symptoms suggestive of a dementing illness, it is important to establish at the outset that the diagnosis really is dementia. Psychiatric illness in elderly patients, particularly depression, may at times be difficult to distin-

Table 30.1   Causes of dementia

Common	Less common
Alzheimer's disease	Hypothyroidism
Multi-infarct dementia	B_{12} deficiency
	Neurosyphilis
	Chronic subdural haematoma
	Frontal lobe neoplasm
	Hydrocephalus
	Chronic alcoholism
	Multiple sclerosis
	Creutzfeldt-Jakob disease
	Huntington's disease
	Multisystem atrophy
	Repeated head trauma
	Progressive supranuclear palsy

guish from a dementing illness. The patient's own account of his illness is not likely to be reliable and information from his spouse or relatives is invaluable. Clinical tests of higher mental function are described in Chapter 7. These tests should be supplemented by a full psychometric assessment by a clinical psychologist if there is any doubt.

Investigations to exclude a treatable cause for the dementia are summarized in Table 30.2. How actively these investigations are pursued will depend on the age of the patient and the degree of clinical suspicion about the underlying cause. An attempt should be made to come to a definite diagnosis even if no active treatment is possible, as the advice and information given to relatives may differ according to the underlying disease.

SPECIFIC CAUSES OF DEMENTIA

Alzheimer's disease

Overall this is the commonest cause of dementia. A distinction was previously made between the presenile and the senile forms of the disease depending whether the onset was before or after the age of 65. It is now recognized that the diseases are pathologically identical and that separation by age of onset is arbitrary. Estimates of the frequency of dementia in community-based studies of elderly populations have established that between 5% and 10% of all people over the age of 70 are significantly demented. Over half of these cases are due to Alzheimer's disease.

Table 30.2 Investigation of dementia

Investigation	Disease to be excluded
Serum vitamin B$_{12}$ concentration	Vitamin B$_{12}$ deficiency
Thyroid function tests	Hypothyroidism
Serum VDRL and TPHA	Neurosyphilis
CT brain scan	Frontal lobe tumour Chronic subdural haematoma
Intraventricular pressure monitoring	Hydrocephalus

Aetiology

Infection by slow viruses or prions, a genetic trait (autosomal dominant with variable penetrance) and a toxic effect of metals, particularly aluminium, have all been suggested as possible causes of Alzheimer's disease. Despite much research, no strong evidence in favour of any one of these has yet emerged.

Pathology

There is severe neuronal loss in the frontal and temporal lobes of the cerebral cortex and in those areas of brain where the diffuse cholinergic and adrenergic projections to the cortex originate—the basal forebrain nuclei and the nucleus of the locus coeruleus respectively. The major neurotransmitter abnormality is a profound reduction in cortical concentrations of acetyl choline and the synthetic enzyme choline acetyltransferase, but reduction in levels of several other cortical neurotransmitters has also been found. The most striking histological abnormalities are senile plaques—extracellular deposits of amyloid protein surrounded by a web of degenerating nerve terminals, which are found in the cerebral cortex and neurofibrillary tangles, and intracellular inclusions of protein filaments, which are found mainly in the pyramidal cells of the cerebral cortex and in the neurones of the basal forebrain nuclei and the thalamus.

Clinical features

The disease is rare before the sixth decade but becomes increasingly common with advancing age. It presents as a slowly progressive dementia. Dysphasia and apraxia are common features of more advanced disease but otherwise focal neurological signs are absent. Epilepsy is unusual except in the very late stages. The average length of survival from diagnosis is less than 5 years.

Treatment

Cholinergic drugs and precursors of acetyl choline, given in an attempt to remedy the major neurotransmitter deficit, have shown disappointing results when assessed in controlled trials. At present, support for the patient's family and long-term institutional care when the patient can no longer be looked after at home are all that can be offered.

Multi-infarct dementia

Multiple cerebral infarction occurs in a setting of widespread arteriosclerotic disease of small cerebral blood vessels. The clinical features of this type of cerebrovascular disease differ from those found when the large arteries are diseased. Occlusion of a major cerebral artery causes infarction of a large amount of brain and there is a correspondingly large neurological deficit. When a small perforating artery is occluded neurological symptoms are often much more subtle. This is hardly surprising; the volume of infarcted brain is many times smaller and the remaining brain has a much greater chance of being able to compensate. However, if the process of occlusion of small arteries continues, multiple small infarcts, usually situated deep in the white matter of the brain, appear. Although the infarcted tissue is not concentrated in one site, the total volume of damaged brain becomes significant. The clinical manifestations of multiple infarction include dementia.

Aetiology and pathology

The most important known predisposing factor for multiple cerebral infarction is systemic hypertension. Untreated, hypertension leads to degenerative changes in the media of small blood vessels and a reduction in the diameter of the lumen. Occlusion of these diseased vessels results in a small localized area of infarction. Because the vascular pathology is generalized many small vessels are at risk of occlusion and, consequently, the infarcts are often multiple.

Clinical features

The presenting features of multiple cerebral infarction depend on the distribution of the infarcts but the typical picture is of a patient with a slow shuffling gait, mild parkinsonian features and deteriorating intellect. Epilepsy is not uncommon and examination often reveals focal neurological signs. Sometimes there is a history of a stepwise progression of the condition to hint at the underlying pathology of multiple small strokes. In other cases gradual loss of memory and deterioration of intellect occur and it may be difficult to distinguish multi-infarct dementia from Alzheimer's disease on the clinical features alone.

Investigation by CT scanning may reveal the presence of small areas of low density, lacunes, within the brain substance. These areas represent the site of infarction.

Treatment

By the time the condition is diagnosed the pathological changes in the blood vessels and the brain itself are far advanced. Control of hypertension is a priority, but care is necessary to avoid reducing systolic blood pressure too far. Overtreatment of blood pressure may actually exacerbate the condition because, in chronic hypertension, the autoregulatory mechanisms controlling cerebral blood flow have been reset for a raised perfusion pressure. Too great a reduction of systolic pressure will result in underperfusion of the brain. The value of anticoagulants and antiplatelet treatment is unproven and currently there is no sound evidence that vasodilators are of benefit.

Creutzfeldt-Jakob disease

This is a very rare disease whose clinical features include myoclonus and relentlessly progressive dementia. It can be transmitted to animals by inoculating them with brain from affected patients but the infectious agent has not so far been isolated. There are a few tragic cases on record in which the disease has been transmitted to other humans by inadequately sterilized surgical instruments during neurosurgical procedures.

Huntington's disease

This is an autosomally dominant inherited condition in which a progressive dementia is combined with involuntary movements. It is dealt with in more detail in Chapter 18.

Hypothyroidism

Slowing of mental processes is a common feature of hypothyroidism. Rarely the mental changes may amount to dementia. The importance of the disease is that it can be treated successfully if the diagnosis is made early.

Neurosyphilis

Neurosyphilis is now a very rare cause of dementia but the diagnosis should always be considered because, of course, it is treatable. The underlying pathology of tertiary syphilis is a chronic, usually basal, meningitis and an obliterative endarteritis. Serological tests for syphilis are positive in the blood in only about two-thirds of cases of neurosyphilis, so if there is a strong suspicion of syphilis as the cause of dementia the CSF must also be examined. The VDRL test on CSF is almost invariably positive in cases of active cerebral disease.

Normal pressure hydrocephalus

The paradoxical term normal pressure hydrocephalus is used to describe a condition of ventricular dilatation not caused by any obstruction of the outflow of CSF from the ventricular system and in which there is no increase in mean CSF pressure. The condition is often idiopathic but may sometimes be the sequel to subarachnoid haemorrhage or basal meningitis. The pathogenesis is not well understood, but studies of CSF hydrodynamics have shown a reduction in CSF absorptive capacity in these patients. Investigation by continuous recording of intracranial pressure reveals that, although mean CSF pressure is normal, there are periods of intermittently raised pressure.

The clinical features are dementia, disturbance of gait and urinary incontinence.

In some patients the insertion of a ventriculo-peritoneal or ventriculo-atrial CSF shunt produces a striking improvement.

Chronic alcoholism

Chronic alcohol abuse, particularly on a background of inadequate nutrition, may lead to a syndrome of dementia. Causation is probably multifactorial involving repeated head trauma, the direct neurotoxic effects of alcohol and the neurological complications of thiamine deficiency.

31. Congenital disorders

CEREBRAL PALSY

The term cerebral palsy was invented to describe a group of non-progressive disorders of motor function, present from birth but, because of the limited range of motor activity of the neonate, often not fully manifested until later in childhood. The aetiology is by no means fully understood. Prematurity, birth trauma and anoxia, and metabolic disturbance in the neonatal period are likely factors in some cases.

Three types of cerebral palsy are recognized.

Spastic cerebral palsy

In this condition the corticospinal pathways are mainly affected. Spasticity and weakness are the predominant features and the child is slow to reach the usual developmental motor milestones. Commonly, the lower limbs are more severely affected than the upper limbs and the term *spastic diplegia* is used to describe the condition. Less common forms of spastic cerebral palsy are spastic tetraplegia, in which the arms and sometimes the bulbar muscles are also affected, and spastic hemiplegia in which one leg and the ipsilateral arm is affected.

Athetoid cerebral palsy

Unilateral or bilateral involuntary movements of athetoid or choreiform type characterize this condition. Pathologically, the basal ganglia show profound loss of neurones. The disorder was previously a common sequel to the severe and prolonged jaundice—kernicterus—that occurred when the fetus was affected by haemolytic disease of the newborn as a result of rhesus iso-immunization.

275

Ataxic cerebral palsy

A combination of ataxia, hypotonia and nystagmus occur as a result of malformation of the cerebellum or a failure of its normal development.

Although these types of cerebral palsy have been depicted as separate entities, they may overlap or coexist. In the more severely affected cases there may be additional problems of mental retardation. Epilepsy often complicates the hemiplegic form of spastic cerebral palsy.

ARNOLD-CHIARI MALFORMATION

The Arnold-Chiari malformation is an abnormality of the position of the lowest part of the medulla and cerebellar tonsils which are displaced downward through the foramen magnum into the upper part of the spinal canal. It may be associated with other defects and developmental abnormalities of the base of the skull and cervical spine: basilar impression of the cervical spine into the skull base, Klippel-Feil syndrome, meningocele or syringomyelia.

The most severe forms present in infancy with hydrocephalus and lower cranial nerve palsies. Milder forms present because of an associated abnormality—often syringomyelia—or with ataxia, a slowly progressive paraparesis or with lower cranial nerve palsies. The presentation may be delayed into adult life.

KLIPPEL-FEIL SYNDROME

This developmental abnormality of the cervical spine consists of the fusion of two or more cervical vertebrae, most commonly C2 and C3. As already noted, it may coexist with other developmental abnormalities. There may be shortening of the neck but often the condition is asymptomatic and only diagnosed when X-rays of the cervical spine are taken.

DYSRAPHISM

Dysraphism describes a group of developmental abnormalities resulting from the failure of complete fusion of the neural tube or the associated bony elements during fetal life. Babies born with the most severe forms, anencephaly and large meningo-encephaloceles, do not survive longer than a few days. Less severe defects can sometimes be repaired surgically but long-term problems of hydrocephalus, poor sphincter control and weakness and spasticity of the lower limbs often cause major disability in later life.

The mildest form of dysraphism is *spina bifida occulta*. This is a failure of closure of the vertebral arch of one or more vertebrae usually in the lumbar spine. There is no cutaneous defect, although occasionally a tuft of hair is present on the overlying skin. Often the condition is asymptomatic, but in some cases there are associated abnormalities within the spinal canal such as lipomas, dermoid cysts or fibrous bands constricting the cauda equina. These may present in childhood or adult life with back pain, sphincter disturbance and neurological defects in the lower limbs.

NEUROCUTANEOUS SYNDROMES

Both skin and neural tissue are derived embryologically from ectoderm and there are a group of developmental disorders gathered under the heading of neurocutaneous syndromes whose clinical features predominantly involve these two tissues.

Tuberose sclerosis

This disorder may be inherited as an autosomal dominant trait, but many cases are sporadic. Small sclerotic lumps of glial tissue, tubers, are found in the cerebral cortex and in the walls of the cerebral ventricles. They have a tendency to calcify and are sometimes visible on a plain skull X-ray.

The cutaneous manifestations are adenoma sebaceum—small raised pink papules looking like warts—found around the nasolabial folds and over the nose and cheeks, depigmented patches, known as ash-leaf patches because of their size and shape, found mainly on the trunk and limbs, and subungual fibromata.

The severity of the condition varies greatly but it is commonly associated with epilepsy and mental subnormality.

Neurofibromatosis

This disorder is also inherited as an autosomal dominant trait. Multiple organ system involvement occurs but the most striking abnormalities are usually in the skin and peripheral nerves.

The common skin manifestations are café au lait patches—light brown patches with a well demarcated outline, variable in size and shaped like a stain of spilt liquid—and mollusca fibrosa—pedunculated skin swellings located mainly on the trunk.

Multiple neurofibromata arise on peripheral nerves. When they lie superficially they can be seen and felt as small, hard, raised lumps. Neurofibromata can also arise on cranial nerves and peripheral nerve roots. The condition is associated with the development of optic nerve gliomas, meningiomas and astrocytomas of the spinal cord.

A separate type of the disorder exists in which bilateral acoustic neuromas occur with great frequency. In affected families these tumours are inherited in an autosomal dominant pattern with very high penetrance. The risk of these tumours developing in the child of an affected parent approaches 50% and it is important that those at risk are kept under regular review by a neurologist.

Sturge-Weber syndrome

This condition consists of a diffuse capillary angioma of the meninges over part of one hemisphere, usually the parietal or occipital lobe, in association with a large port-wine facial naevus within the cutaneous distribution of the trigeminal nerve. In the majority of cases there is an accompanying congenital abnormality of the eye on the affected side.

The cortex underlying the angioma is abnormal and contains areas of calcification which may be visible on a skull X-ray. There is often a contralateral hemiparesis or homonymous visual field defect and epilepsy is very common.

32. Drug-induced disease of the nervous system

A large number of the drugs in current medical use may have adverse effects that involve the nervous system. Patients should always be asked whether they are taking drugs prescribed by other medical practitioners, or if they are taking any proprietary medication on their own initiative.

Few of us possess memories tenacious enough to remember the adverse effects of all the commonly prescribed drugs. Set out in Table 32.1 is a list of some of the drugs which can cause disturbance of neurological function.

Table 32.1 Adverse effects of drugs on the nervous system

Adverse effect	Drug
Seizures	Tricyclic antidepressants
	Chlorpromazine
	Amphetamines
Tremor	Lithium
	Sodium valproate
Involuntary movementss	L-Dopa
	Phenothiazines
	Butyrophenones
VIII nerve damage	Gentamicin
	Streptomycin
	Other aminoglycoside antibiotics
Optic nerve damage	Chloroquine
	Ethambutol
Peripheral neuropathy	Isoniazid
	Vincristine
	Metronidazole
	Dapsone
Myasthenia	Penicillamine
	Aminoglycoside antibiotics

Table 32.1 *(cont'd)*

Adverse effect	Drug
Myopathy	Steroids
Cerebellar syndrome	Phenytoin
Acute confusional state	Corticosteroids Benzhexol and other anticholinergics L-Dopa Isoniazid Bismuth

Further Reading

NEUROANATOMY
Fitzgerald M J T 1985 Neuroanatomy basic and applied. Baillière Tindall, London
   If you need to check up on neuroanatomy try this readable and excellently illustrated book.

NEUROPHYSIOLOGY
Carpenter R H S 1984 Neurophysiology. Edward Arnold, London
Stein J F 1982 An introduction to neurophysiology. Blackwell Scientific Publications, Oxford
   These two books explain current views of the physiology of the nervous system in a clear and interesting way.

NEUROPSYCHOLOGY
Graham Beaumont J 1983 Introduction to neuropsychology. Blackwell Scientific Publications, Oxford
   This book is recommended to anyone wanting to find out more about higher cortical functions.

CLINICAL NEUROLOGY
Lindsay K W, Bone I, Callander R 1986 Neurology and neurosurgery illustrated. Churchill Livingstone, Edinburgh
   An excellent account of clinical neurology, written mainly for postgraduates but valuable for medical students too.
Walton Sir J 1985 Brain's diseases of the nervous system, 9th edn. Oxford University Press, Oxford
   The classic reference book to consult for detailed descriptions of neurological diseases.
Spillane J D 1982 An atlas of clinical neurology, 3rd edn. Oxford University Press, Oxford
   A superbly illustrated book of diseases of the nervous system.
Aids to the examination of peripheral nerve injuries. 1986 Baillière Tindall, London
   This short book provides details of how to examine patients with peripheral nerve injuries.

Index